Recent Results in Cancer Research 101

AF774220

Recent Results in Cancer Research

Volume 95: Spheroids in Cancer Research
Edited by H. Acker, J. Carlsson, R. Durand, R. M. Sutherland
1984. 83 figures, 12 tables. IX, 183. ISBN 3-540-13691-6

Volume 96: Adjuvant Chemotherapy of Breast Cancer
Edited by H.-J. Senn
1984. 98 figures, 91 tables. X, 243. ISBN 3-540-13738-6

Volume 97: Small Cell Lung Cancer
Edited by S. Seeber
1985. 44 figures, 47 tables. VII, 166. ISBN 3-540-13798-X

Volume 98: Perioperative Chemotherapy
Edited by U. Metzger, F. Largiadèr, H.-J. Senn
1985. 48 figures, 45 tables. XII, 157. ISBN 3-540-15124-9

Volume 99: Peptide Hormones in Lung Cancer
Edited by K. Havemann, G. Sorenson, C. Gropp
1985. 100 figures, 63 tables. XII, 248. ISBN 3-540-15504-X

Volume 100: Therapeutic Strategies in Primary and Metastatic Liver Cancer
Edited by C. Herfarth, P. Schlag, P. Hohenberger
1986. 163 figures, 104 tables. ISBN 3-540-16011-6

Locoregional High-Frequency Hyperthermia and Temperature Measurement

Edited by
G. Bruggmoser, W. Hinkelbein, R. Engelhardt,
and M. Wannenmacher

With 96 Figures and 8 Tables

Springer-Verlag
Berlin Heidelberg New York Tokyo

Dipl. Phys. G. Bruggmoser
Dr. W. Hinkelbein
Prof. Dr. R. Engelhardt
Prof. Dr. Dr. M. Wannenmacher

Abteilung für Röntgen- und Strahlentherapie
im Zentrum Radiologie, Universitätsklinik
Hugstetter Strasse 55, 7800 Freiburg i. Brsg., FRG

ISBN-13: 978-3-642-82532-3 e-ISBN-13: 978-3-642-82530-9
DOI: 10.1007/978-3-642-82530-9

Library of Congress Cataloging-in-Publication Data. Main entry under title: Locoregional high-frequency hyperthermia and temperature measurement. (Recent results in cancer research; 101) Proceedings of a workshop. Includes bibliographies and index.
1. Cancer-Radiotherapy-Congresses. 2. Thermotherapy-Congresses. 3. Thermometers and thermometry-Congresses. I. Bruggmoser, G. (Gregor), 1948-. II. Series. [DNLM:
1. Hyperthermia, Induced-methods-congresses. 2. Neoplasms-therapy-congresses.
WI RE106P v. 101/QZ 266 L819] RC261.R35 vol. 101 616.99'4 s [616.99'40632] 85-22082
[RC271.T5]

Typesetting: Appl, Wemding
2125/3140-543210

Preface

The present challenge in the treatment of tumors is to reduce the number of patients that still die as a result of primary tumors. Today, the percentage of such deaths remains high at 30%, even when all the common therapeutic methods, namely surgery, radiotherapy, and chemotherapy, are applied.

In order to reduce this percentage, new types of radiation sources with a higher linear energy transfer have been introduced, such as neutrons and pions. Fractionation patterns have been modified and radiosensitizers have been applied to increase biological efficiency. Studies of the combined application of chemotherapy and radiotherapy have been made to find the best therapeutic effect.

In the early 1970s biological findings confirmed the effect of hyperthermia on tumor cells. The first clinical studies on hyperthermia treatment demonstrated that it resulted in better local tumor control. Further application of this treatment modality showed that hyperthermia should be used in addition to radiotherapy and chemotherapy.

Despite these encouraging results, hyperthermia has not been introduced into common clinical use, due primarily to technical problems. There are a number of methods of transferring heat into tumors; however, with regard to physical conditions, an optimum method has not yet been found. One of the reasons is that up to now we have had no reliable method of obtaining thermal mapping of all parts of the human body. Such measurements are required not only for dosimetric purposes but also for the regulation of a hyperthermic system.

The main objective of this volume is to provide a realistic survey of the methods presently available in the area of high-frequency temperature measurement and computer-assisted calculations.

Physicians, medical physicists, and representatives from private industry - all of whom are working in this field - have been invited to a workshop to discuss the technical and physical problems of hyperthermia. The workshop was intended to take on a more informative character: The clinicians presented their requirements in detail so that the physicists know exactly and in detail what technical problems they are being asked to solve.

Freiburg, October 1985 M. Wannenmacher

Contents

*List of Contributors**

* The address of the principal author is given on the first page of each contribution

1 Page on which contribution begins

Clinical Requirements

Clinical Requirements of Local and Regional Hyperthermia Application

R. Engelhardt

Universitätsklinik Freiburg, Medizinische Klinik, Hugstetter Strasse 55, 7800 Freiburg i. Brsg., FRG

Hyperthermia is on the way to becoming a useful tool for the treatment of patients with cancer. This optimistic point of view is based on the following biological findings:

1. Heat is cytotoxic in a number of malignant cells at temperatures above 42.5 °C (Gerner et al. 1975)
2. Heat increases the effectiveness of ionizing radiation by both sensitization and synergism, especially at hypoxic conditions in S-phase cells and at low pH (Gerweck et al. 1983; Overgaard 1982; Westra and Dewey 1971)
3. Heat enhances the effect of several cytotoxic drugs, even at temperatures below 42.5 °C in some cases. Low pH seems to increase the enhancement (Hahn and Shiu 1983)

These data provide the rationale for taking different approaches to the clinical application of heat as a cancer treatment modality:

1. Cell-killing by heat alone
2. Cell-killing by heat combined with radiation
3. Cell-killing by heat combined with chemotherapy

Cell-Killing by Heat Alone

The temperature level needed in this case (42.5 °C or above) is not tolerable on a whole-body scale. The approach, therefore, is restricted to local or regional application. Its effectiveness is enhanced by a milieu characterized by a low pH, nutrient depletion, and hypoxia, which are often found in solid tumors. Heat alone could therefore be especially useful in treating bulky disease.

Several groups have reported on their results of heat treatment for tumors in men (Hahn 1982) (see Table 1). Superficially localized tumors were treated by ultrasound heating. Both remission rate and duration of remission increased with rising temperature (43° up to 50 °C). However, permanent cure is rare for the following reasons:

1. Heat distribution within the tumor is not homogeneous and thus "cold spots" occur where the heat is not high enough to kill all the cells completely.
2. Heterogeneity is mainly due to the nonuniform perfusion of the lesion.
3. There is particularly good vascularization in the tumor bed and a large amount of proliferating tumor cells.

Recent Results in Cancer Research. Vol 101

Table 1. Results of ultrasound local hyperthermia (Hahn 1982)

Institution	Temperature (°C)	Evaluable courses	Responses (complete and partial)	%	Median duration of response
Stanford	43 -44	23	9	39	6 weeks
M. D. Anderson Hospital and Tumor Institute	43 -44	15	8	53	29 days
Stanford	44.1-45	21	10	48	6 weeks
M. D. Anderson Hospital and Tumor Institute	45 -47	7	3	43	45 days
M. D. Anderson Hospital and Tumor Institute	48 -50	6	5	83	250 days

Table 2. Heat resistance of normal tissues

Tissue	Animal	Temperature	Time	Reference
Skin	Pig	45 °C	1 h	Henriques (1947)
	Human			Martinez et al. (1980)
Muscle	Pig	45 °C	½ h	Martinez et al. (1980)
Fat				
Cartilage	Rat	44 °C	1 h	Field (1978)
Brain	Mouse	42 °C	1 h	Gwozda et al. (1978)

In areas with high perfusion rates, the heat itself and the factors promoting the heat effect (low pH, low O_2, low nutrient concentration) are less pronounced and cell-kill remains incomplete. Furthermore, the shape of a tumor is usually irregular with poorly defined borders. The heated volume, therefore, has to include a safety margin within the adjacent normal tissue. Both the temperature level and the duration of heating (heat dose) are therefore limited by the heat tolerance of the normal adjacent tissue.

Although studies have indicated that some tumor cells are more sensitive to heat than their normal counterparts (Giovanella et al. 1979), this is of limited clinical significance. Tumors, especially metastatic tumors, are mostly surrounded by tissues completely different from those the tumors are derived from. Consequently, the selectivity of the heat effect has to be defined for each individual tumor by comparing its sensitivity to heat with the most heat-sensitive tissue adjacent to the tumor. The heat tolerance for some normal tissues has been determined in humans and animals (see Table 2).

In summary, the therapeutic efficiency of heat alone is defined by:

1. The intrinsic heat sensitivity of the tumor cells and the degree of heterogeneity of the tumor cells in this respect (Rofstad 1984)
2. The degree of inhomogeneity within the single lesion in terms of perfusion rate and milieu factors
3. The shape and architecture of the border of the lesions
4. The heat sensitivity of the most sensitive adjacent normal tissue(s)

5. The topographical situation of the lesion (depth, physical properties of the surrounding tissue, etc.)

Some of the limitations accounting for the clinical failure of treating tumors by heat alone may be overcome by combining heat with radiation therapy or chemotherapy.

Cell-Killing by Heat Combined with Radiation

The reasoning for combining heat with irradiation is mainly based on their synergism (Dewey 1984; Overgaard 1982):

1. Hypoxic cells, which are highly radioresistant, are killed by heat as efficiently as well-oxygenated ones.
2. Late S-phase cells, which are radioresistant, are highly thermosensitive.
3. Thermal enhancement of the X-ray effect takes place at temperatures well below the cytotoxic level (40 °C in melanoma cells) (Streffer et al. 1984).
4. Heat is thought to have a dose modification factor of 1.3. This means that it takes about 30% less radiation to obtain the same cell-kill when heat is added (Westra and Dewey 1971).

Several clinical studies have demonstrated the effect of hyperthermia in combination with radiation therapy with respect to improved response rates (Kim and Hahn 1979; Kim et al. 1978; Sauer 1984). But due to the lack of standardized heating techniques and temperature measurement devices, the results are not comparable. The most conclusive and the only randomized trial was performed in dogs (Dewhirst et al. 1984). The efficacy of the combination was clearly dependent on the lowest temperature measured in the tumor under treatment, which demonstrates the importance of the homogeneity of heating.

Cell-Killing by Heat Combined with Chemotherapy

Heat is able to enhance the effect of chemotherapeutic drugs. This is due to the different effects of heat, which are exerted both at the tumor level and at the cellular level. As mentioned above, heat is more effective in poorly vascularized areas, whereas the effect of chemotherapy is dependent on effective blood perfusion. The two modes of therapy therefore complement one another. When the blood flow increases during heat treatment, the synergistic effect becomes even more pronounced. Since blood flow tends to stop after 30 min of heating at 43 °C, the timing of heat and drug application must be considered an important aspect in clinical treatments.

Even more attractive is the fact that heat can increase the cell-killing ability of many drugs. From experiments in cell lines and in animal tumors, three types of drug-heat interaction have been described (Hahn 1982):

1. Drugs enhanced linearly by increasing temperature
2. Drugs enhanced only above a threshold temperature of about 43 °C
3. Drugs cytotoxic only at elevated temperatures

Although increasingly more information is accumulating from in vitro studies on human tumor cells to suggest that there may be exceptions to this classification (Kano et al. 1984; Neumann et al. 1984a), it can nevertheless be used as a guide for the discussion of the possible applications of thermochemotherapy in man.

1. Drugs that become enhanced or cytotoxic at temperatures as low as 39°-42 °C are suitable not only for localized regional but also for whole-body application (Engelhardt 1984; Engelhardt et al. 1983). In this case, the question of the selectivity of the thermal enhancement has to be answered by comparing the degree of enhancement of the toxic side effects.
   As has been published elsewhere (Neumann et al. 1984a, b), our group has demonstrated in vitro that there are human tumors in which the effect of several drugs can be enhanced considerably more than in human bone marrow progenitor cells. In these experiments, using a modified clonogenic assay at 37 °C and at 40.5 °C, a marked tumor-to-drug-related individuality was demonstrated, which indicates a broad spectrum of possible reactions.
2. When drugs that are enhanced only above a threshold temperature of 42 °C are used, heat must be applied regionally. In this case, the drug may be adminstered systemically or regionally, but the thermal enhancement is restricted to the heated volume. There is no enhancement of the systemic toxicity, which is certainly an advantage.
3. Finally, there is a group of drugs which are characterized by having no cytoxicity at 37 °C but becoming potent cell inactivators at elevated temperatures. Such a mode of action has been described for a number of sulfhydryl-rich compounds (Kapp and Hahn 1979) [cysteamine, cystrine and AET (2-aminoethylisothiourium bromide)], naturally occurring polyamines (Gerner et al. 1980) (e.g., putrescine, spermidine, and spermine), and amphotericin B. Similar effects have been observed for ethanol and some local anesthetics (Li et al. 1980) (e.g., lidocaine and procaine), which act by inducing temperature shifts. Again the combination of these drugs with regional hyperthermia would be of special clinical interest.

The combination of regionally restricted drug administration and regional heating has been used for isolated limb perfusion. Some groups (Cavaliere et al. 1982; Stehlin et al. 1984) have found this technique to have beneficial effects in patients with malignant melanomas and sarcomas. But definitive confirmation of the therapeutic advantage of this approach still has to be established in randomized trials.

Regional drug administration has become an area of increasing interest during the past years (Ensminger and Gyves 1984). Combining this approach with regional percutaneous heating seems to offer another attractive possibility for the heat-drug combination. The preliminary results seem promising, although controlled, prospective, and even randomized trials are still unavailable (Falk 1984; Storm and Morton 1983).

In summary, numerous biological studies carried out over the past decade have established the rationale for the use of (1) heat alone, (2) heat in combination with radiation, and (3) heat in combination with cytostatic drugs in cancer therapy.

But although heat has all these advantages, hyperthermia is only slowly being adopted as a treatment of cancer. This is primarily due to the technical difficulty of heating tumors to appropriate temperatures and determining the temperature distribution obtained.

Both uniform heating and temperature measurement are hampered by the wide variety of tissues within a given volume to be heated. These tissues have different characteristics in terms of energy absorption, depending on the type of heating energy used. The tumors are mostly irregular in shape, size, and site and are usually not sharply separated from the surrounding normal tissue. Vascularization and perfusion rates of tumors are not uniform and often change during heating. But clearly the controlled uniform heating of an arbitrary volume is essential to induce cytotoxicity or enhancement effects safely. Areas of undertreatment in the tumor will otherwise lead to the survival of an unknown number of tumor cells, which will cause growth of the tumor and hence treatment failure. "Hot spots," on the other hand, may lead to damage of normal tissue.

For nonlinear cell-killing with respect to temperature, an accuracy of 1 °C is the minimum requirement for both the safety of treatment and the prevention of side effects.

References

Cavaliere R, DiFilippo F, Morrica G, Santori F, Varanese A, Pantano FP, Cassanelli A, Aloe L, Monticelli G (1982) Hyperthermic perfusion for treatment of tumors of the extremities. Chemioterapia 1: 278-287

Dewey WC (1984) Inactivation of mammalian cells by combined hyperthermia and radiation. Front Radiat Ther Oncol 18: 29-40

Dewhirst MW, Sim DA, Grochowski KJ (1984) Thermal influence on radiation induced complications vs. tumor response in a phase III randomized trial. In: Overgaard J (ed) Hyperthermic oncology. Taylor and Francis, London, pp 313-316 (Summary papers, vol 1)

Engelhardt R (1985) Whole-body-hyperthermia. Methods and clinical results. In: Overgaard J (ed) Hyperthermic oncology, vol 2. Taylor and Francis, London, pp 263-276

Engelhardt R, Neumann H, Hinkelbein W, Adam G, Weth R, Löhr GW (1984) Clinical studies in thermo-chemotherapy. In: Engelhardt R, Wallach DH (eds) Hyperthermia. In: Spitzy KH, Karrer K (editors) Proceedings of the 13th International Congress of Chemotherapy, Vienna 1983, vol 18. Egermann, Vienna, pp 273/41-273/46

Ensminger WD, Gyves JW (1984) Regional cancer chemotherapy. Cancer Treat Rep 68: 101-115

Falk RE (1984) Possibilities and value of hyperthermia in combined modality treatment (Abstr). Conference on Therapeutic Strategies in Primary and Metastatic Liver Cancer, Heidelberg, Sept 17-19, 1984

Field SB (1978) The response of normal tissues to hyperthermia alone or in combination with x-rays. In: Streffer C, van Beuningen D, Dietzel F, Roettinger E, Robinson JE, Scherer E, Seeber S, Trott KR (eds) Cancer therapy by hyperthermia and radiation. Urban and Schwarzenberg, Munich, pp 37-48

Gerner EW, Connor WG, Boone MCM, Doss JD, Mayer EG, Miller RG (1975) The potential of localized heating as adjunct to radiation therapy. Radiology 119: 715-720

Gerner EW, Cress A, Stickney D, Holmes D, Culver P (1980) Factors regulating membrane permeability alter thermal resistance. Ann NY Acad Sci 335: 215-233

Gerweck LE, Dahlberg WK, Greco B (1983) Effect of pH on single or fractionated heat treatments at 42-45 degrees. Cancer Res 43: 1163-1167

Giovanella BC, Stehlin JS, Morgan AC (1979) Selective lethal effects of supranormal temperatures on human neoplastic cells. Cancer Res 39: 2236-2241

Gwozda B, Dyduch A, Gryber H, Paus B (1978) Structural changes in brain mitochondria of mice subjected to hyperthermia. Exp Pathol 15: 124-126

Hahn GM (1982) Hyperthermia and cancer. Plenum, New York

Hahn GM, Shiu EC (1983) Effect of pH and elevated temperatures on the cytotoxicity of some chemotherapeutic agents on chinese hamster cells in vitro. Cancer Res 43: 5789-5791

Henriques FC Jr (1947) Studies on thermal injury. Arch Pathol 43: 489-502

Kano E, Furukawa M, Yoshikawa S, Tsubouchi S, Kondo T, Sugahara T (1984) Hyperthermic chemopotentiation and chemical thermosensitization. In: Overgaard J (ed) Hyperthermic oncology vol 1. Taylor and Francis, London, pp 437-440

Kapp DS, Hahn GM (1979) Thermosensitization by sulfhydryl compounds of exponentially growing Chinese hamster cells. Cancer Res 39: 4630-4635

Kim JH, Hahn EW (1979) Clinical and biological studies of localized hyperthermia. Cancer Res 39: 2258-2261

Kim JH, Hahn EW, Tokita N (1978) Combination hyperthermia and radiation therapy for cutaneous malignant melanoma. Cancer 41: 2143-2148

Li GC, Shiu EC, Hahn GM (1980) Similarities in cellular inactivation by hyperthermia or by ethanol. Radiat Res 82: 257-268

Martinez A, Kernahan P, Prionas S, Hahn GM (1980) The effects of radiofrequency heating in normal fat and muscular tissues. A histological based tissue injury grading system. In: Dethlefsen LA (ed) Proceedings of the Third International Symposium on Cancer Therapy by Hyperthermia, Drugs and Radiation. Fort Collins, Colorado, USA, p 132 (Abstract TIII 33)

Neumann HA, Fiebig HH, Löhr GW, Engelhardt R (1984a) Combined hyperthermic and cytostatic treatment of human bone marrow progenitors and human tumor cells (Abstr). 4th International Symposium on Hyperthermic Oncology, Aarhus, Denmark, July 2-6, 1984

Neumann HA, Fiebig HH, Löhr GW, Engelhardt R (1984b) Effects of cytostatic drugs and 40.5 °C hyperthermia on human clonogenic tumor cells. Eur J Cancer, to be published

Overgaard J (1982) Can the thermal enhancement ratio be estimated by a simple formula? (Abstr). Strahlentherapie 158: 388

Rofstad EK (1984) Thermotolerance in human melanoma xenografts in vitro and in vivo. In: Overgaard J (ed) Hyperthermic oncology. Taylor and Francis, London, pp 199-202 (Summary papers, vol 1)

Sauer R (1984) Hyperthermie bei Radioresistenz. Klinische Ergebnisse. Beitr Onkol 18: 427-442

Song CW, Kang MS, Rhee JG, Levitt SH (1980) Effect of hyperthermia on vascular function in normal and neoplastic tissues. Ann NY, Acad Sci 335: 35-47

Stehlin JS Jr, Giovanella BC, Gutierrez AE, Ipolyi PD, Greff PJ (1984) 15 year's experience with hyperthermic perfusion for treatment of soft tissue sarcoma and malignant melanoma of the extremities. Front Radiat Ther Oncol 18: 177-182

Storm FK, Morton DL (1983) Hyperthermia: adjunctive modality for hepatic infusion chemotherapy. Semin Oncol 10: 223

Streffer C, van Beuningen D, Devi PU (1984) Hyperthermie in Kombination mit ionisierenden Strahlen in der Behandlung resistenter Tumoren. Beitr Onkol 18: 415-426

Westra A, Dewey WC (1971) Variation in sensitivity to heat shock during cell-cycle of chinese hamster cells in vitro. Int J Radiat Biol 19: 467-477

Field Penetration from Electromagnetic Applicators for Localized Hyperthermia

J. W. Hand and R. H. Johnson

Medical Research Council, Cyclotron Unit Hammersmith Hospital, Ducane Road, London, W12 OHS, United Kingdom

Introduction

When a plane electromagnetic wave propagates through a uniform medium the magnitude of the **E** field is reduced by a factor $1/_e$ in a distance D where

$$D = \frac{c \cdot \sqrt{2}}{\omega \left\{ [\varepsilon'^2 + \{\sigma/\omega\varepsilon_0\}^2]^{1/2} - \varepsilon' \right\}^{1/2}} \qquad (1)$$

and c = velocity of light, ω = angular frequency, ε'^1 = real part of the relative permittivity of the medium, σ = conductivity of the medium, and ε_0 = permittivity of free space. D is known as the (plane wave) penetration depth, and the absorbed power density (proportional to E^2) is reduced to approximately 13.5% within this distance. A closely related parameter is the half-value distance, $d_{1/2}$; this is the distance in which the absorbed power density is reduced by a factor of one-half. The relationship between these parameters is:

$$d_{1/2} = 0.346\, D \qquad (2)$$

It follows from Eq. (1) that plane wave penetration into a medium increases as ω and σ are decreased, and this is illustrated in Fig. 1.

Although the parameters D or $d_{1/2}$ are often used in discussion of electromagnetic heating of tissues, the penetrating ability of practical applicators used to heat inhomogeneous tissues depends strongly on the size of the applicators, the curvature of tissues, and the thickness of tissue layers relative to the wavelength of the electromagnetic field. This paper presents a brief review of field penetration from applicators designed for localized hyperthermia and discusses both the dependence of penetration from a single applicator on the parameters mentioned above and improvements which may be attainable through the use of multiple-applicator systems.

Radiofrequency Applicators

If an applicator is small compared with the wavelength, the electromagnetic fields produced in the tissue tend to be dominated by the near fields, which are very strong close to the applicator but decrease rapidly with increasing distance from it. The effectiveness of such an applicator in heating tissue at depth is considerably less than that predicted using plane wave assumptions. Simple analyses of the **E**-field – (capacitive electrodes) and

Recent Results in Cancer Research. Vol 101

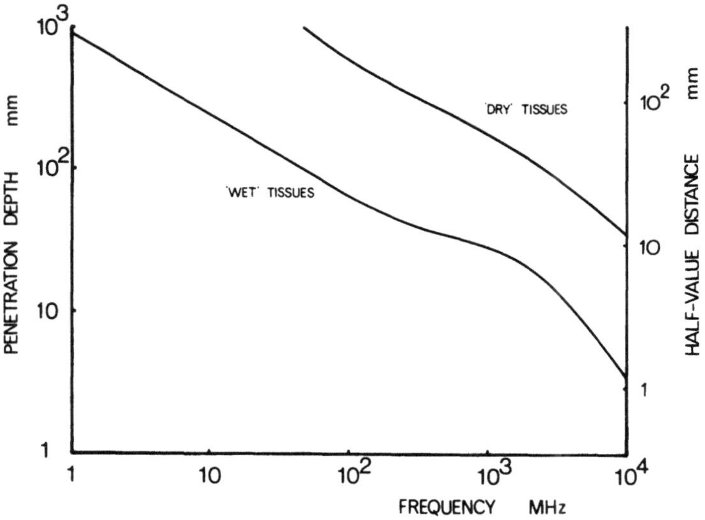

Fig. 1. Plane wave penetration into tissues with high and low water content

H-field - ("pancake" coil) techniques commonly used for radiofrequency-induced hyperthermia (for example, at 13.56 MHz or 27.12 MHz) illustrate this point.

A common arrangement for local heating by radiofrequencies is to place a small electrode (typically less than 5-6 cm in diameter) above the region of interest and to arrange for the patient to lie on a larger, return electrode. Some characteristics of this technique can be seen by considering the simple model of a circular disk, radius *a*, in contact with a uniform medium, as shown in Fig. 2. Since the distances involved are small compared with the wavelength, a quasi static solution is valid. If the disk is at a uniform potential Φ_0 with respect to a second electrode at infinity (in practice the separation between electrodes would be several disk diameters), then the electric field $\mathbf{E}(r, z)$ is given by (e.g., Wiley and Webster 1982):

$$\mathbf{E} = -\nabla \Phi(r, z) \tag{3}$$

where $$\Phi(r, z) = \frac{2\,\Phi_0}{\pi} \sin^{-1}\left\{\frac{2\,a}{[(r-a)^2+z^2]^{1/2}+[(r+a)^2+z^2]^{1/2}}\right\} \text{ for } z \neq 0 \tag{4}$$

and $$\Phi(r, o) = \frac{2\,\Phi_0}{\pi} \sin^{-1}\left\{\frac{r}{a}\right\} \text{ for } r \geqslant a \tag{5}$$

Figure 3 is a plot of $\mathbf{E}(r/a, z/a)$ and shows the large fringing fields at the edge of the disk. The electric field is predominantly perpendicular to the plane of the disk for $r \lesssim 0.7\,a$, and this can lead to excessive heating in the fat regions of fat and muscle layers. In Fig. 4 $E^2(r)/E^2(a, 0.1\,a)$ is shown for several values of z. The absorbed power density is very large close to the edges of the disk and decreases rapidly with increasing distance from the disk. In practice the region close to the disk electrode, say $O < z \lesssim 0.3\,a$, would be contained within a bolus to avoid excessive heating of the tissues under the edge of the disk. Beyond this region the absorbed power density decreases with increasing z with an "effective" penetration depth $\sim a$ (typically less than 3 cm). Local heating by a "pancake coil" may be analyzed by modeling the n turns of the coil as n current carrying, concentric circular loops placed a distance h above layers of fat and muscle tissue (Guy et al. 1971).

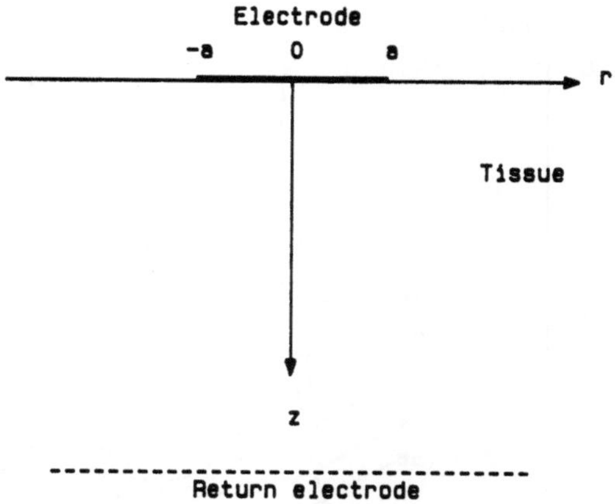

Fig. 2. Circular disk, in contact with uniform medium, and distant return electrode

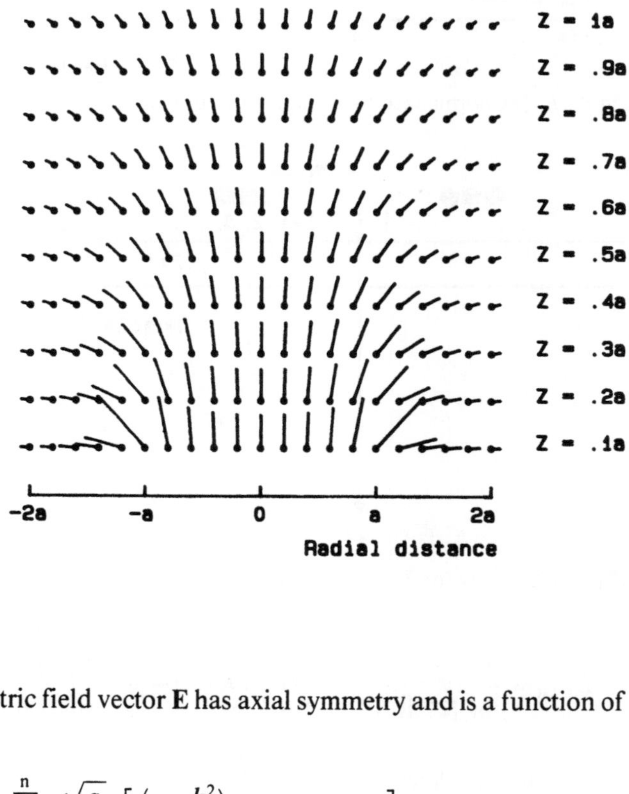

Fig. 3. Electric Field E due to circular electrode of Fig. 2

The magnetically induced electric field vector **E** has axial symmetry and is a function of r and z. The component E_Φ is:

$$E_\Phi = -j\omega \sum_{i=1}^{n} A_{\Phi_i} = -\frac{j\omega\mu_0 I}{\sqrt{r}} \sum_{i=1}^{n} \frac{\sqrt{a_i}}{k_i} \left[\left(1 - \frac{k_i^2}{z}\right) K(k_i) - E(k_i) \right] \tag{6}$$

where $k_i = \dfrac{4\,a_i}{(a_i + r)^2 + z^2}$

A_Φ is the magnetic vector potential, $K(k_i)$ and $E(k_i)$ are the complete elliptical integrals of the first and second kinds, respectively, a_i is the radius of the ith loop, $\omega = 2\,\pi \times$ frequency, and $\mu o = 4\,\pi \times 10^{-7}\ H/\text{m}$. The electric field normal to the tissue surface due to the potential differences between loops and the tissue is approximated by

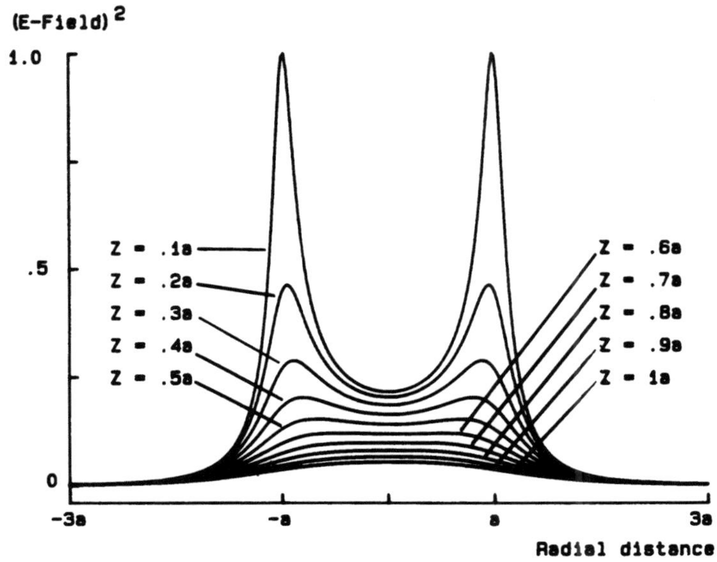

Fig. 4. $E^2(r)$, normalized to $E^2(a, 0.1\,a)$, for several values of z

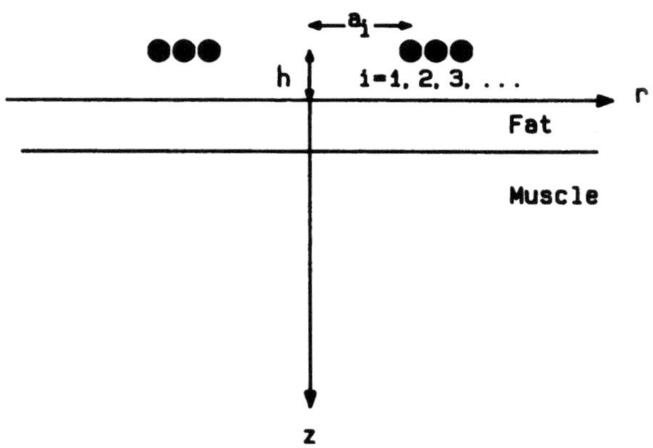

Fig. 5. Geometry for model of pancake coil

$$E_{z,\,\mathrm{fat}} = \frac{1}{\varepsilon_{\mathrm{fat}}} \sum_{i=1}^{n} \frac{-Q_i\,2h}{[(a_i+r)^2+h^2]} \left(K(k_i) - \frac{4\,a_i\,r}{[(r-a_i)^2+h^2]}\,B(k_i)\right) \tag{7}$$

$$\text{with } B(k_i) = K(k_i) - \left[\frac{K(k_i)-E(k_i)}{k_i^2}\right]$$

If each loop is taken to be at a single potential, these potentials can be calculated in terms of the loop inductances. The constants Q_i ($i=1, \ldots, n$) in Eq. 7 are found in terms of these potentials. The absorbed power density is

$$W_{\mathrm{fat}} = \sigma_{\mathrm{fat}}\,[E_\Phi^2 + E_z^2] \tag{8}$$

in the fat. The E_z term is of less importance in the underlying muscle and so

$$W_{\mathrm{muscle}} = \sigma_{\mathrm{muscle}}\,E_\Phi^2 \tag{9}$$

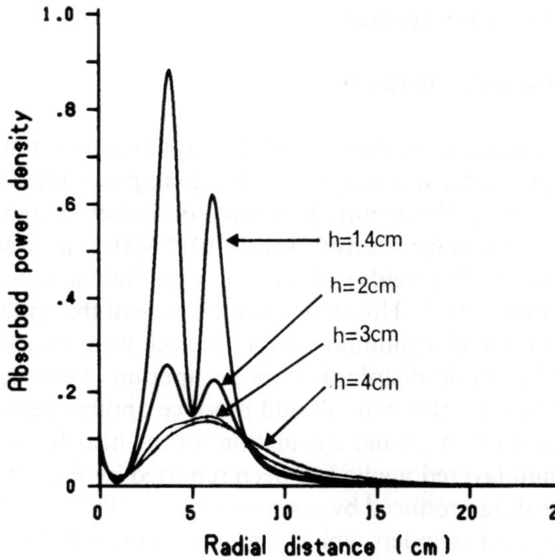

Fig. 6. Normalized absorbed power density at the surface of the fat layer, for four values of h due to a three-turn ($a_1 = 4$ cm, $a_2 = 5$ cm, $a_3 = 6$ cm) 27.12-MHz coil

The radial dependence of absorbed power density at the surface of a 1-cm-thick layer of fat ($z = 0$) (normalized to the respective maximum of absorbed power density in the muscle layer) due to a three-turn coil (radii 4, 5, and 6 cm) driven at 27.12 MHz is shown in Fig. 6. When the separation between coil and tissues (h) is less than about 3 cm, the distribution of absorbed power density is dominated by the effects of the potential distribution around the coil which become strongly dependent upon h when h is small. For example, as h is decreased from $h = 1.4$ cm to $h = 1$ cm, the maximum absorbed power density in the fat layer increases from 0.9 times to 3.9 times that in muscle. For larger values of h ($\gtrsim$ 3 cm), the distribution is dominated by the E_{Φ} component of the electric field. Under these conditions, the effective penetration depth in muscle tissue is typically 3–4 cm, the larger values being achieved with large-diameter coils and/or increased separation between coils and tissue (Hand et al. 1982; Lerch and Kohn 1983).

Morita and Bach Anderson (1982) made an analytical study of near-field coupling of electromagnetic sources to circular cylinders with dielectric properties similar to those of muscle. They considered elementary electric and magnetic dipoles with each of three polarizations relative to the longitudinal axis, spaced at distances much smaller than the free-space wavelength from this axis, at frequencies below 300 MHz for which the wavelengths and plane wave penetration depths in the cylinders were large compared with the radius. Using this long wavelength approximation, they showed that the axially (z-) aligned electric dipole source achieved the greatest penetration, a finding of relevance in the design of applicators for deep heating, while the x- and y-aligned electric dipoles produced distributions of absorbed power which were highly dependent upon the separation between the source and the cylinder. Such dependence was less critical in the case of the y-directed magnetic dipole, and an applicator based on this arrangement has been described by Bach Andersen et al. (1984). The x-directed magnetic dipole produced an absorbed power distribution with zero along that axis, similar to that associated with the plane ("pancake") coil discussed earlier. Near-field fall-off from finite-sized aperture sources, which can be considered as distributions of these elementary sources, is dependent upon aperture size and less rapid than for elementary sources.

Microwave Applicators

Waveguide Applicators

At frequencies above 300 MHz, applicators can be constructed with dimensions comparable with a wavelength, leading to improved radiation efficiency.

Guy (1971) reported an analysis of electromagnetic fields and associated heating due to a rectangular aperture source (915 MHz) in direct contact with plane layers of fat and muscle. The fields in the tissue were evaluated using a Fourier transform technique (Harrington 1961). Hot spots near the edge of the applicator due to the rapidly diverging fields at these discontinuities in the source were clearly identified and it was suggested that a TE_{10} mode distribution on an aperture 1 wavelength (in fat) high and between 1 and 2 wavelengths wide should produce optimal heating in muscle compared with that in the fat layer. A similar calculation for the near fields of a circular applicator irradiating into multilayered media has been reported by Fray et al. (1982). Ho et al. (1971) analyzed the heating produced by aperture sources (433-2450 MHz; TE_{10} mode) in contact with triple-layered cylinders which simulated human limbs. These workers also found that the heating produced in the fat relative to that in muscle was minimized when the height of the aperture was equal to 1 wavelength in the fat region and that excessive heating occurred in the fat when the height of the aperture was less than half the wavelength. In some cases the cylindrical geometry led to standing waves in the muscle region. In another study, Ho (1979) showed that electrically small apertures in contact with tissue equivalent spheres produced a high specific absorption rate (SAR) in superficial regions. The SAR produced at the center of the sphere relative to that at the surface depended on frequency in a resonant manner, with both the resonant frequency and relative heating at the center reduced as the radius of the sphere was increased. For muscle-like spheres with radius greater than about 6 cm, the SAR produced in superficial regions was greater than that produced at the center of the sphere. Source frequencies in the range 10 MHz to 10 GHz were considered in this study.

The field distributions on the electrically small apertures typical of hyperthermia applicators are often approximated by assuming that the aperture is on a perfectly conducting plane in contact with tissue. Turner and Kumar (1982) modeled the aperture fields by an array of Hertzian dipoles and assumed that the field distribution on the aperture was that in the waveguide (TE_{10}). They showed that effective penetration depths associated with apertures having practical dimensions were smaller than plane wave values and that for very small apertures the effective penetration depth was quite sensitive to aperture size. Some results of these calculations are included in Fig. 7. Audet et al. (1980) and Robillard et al. (1980) discussed effective penetration depth for rectangular aperture supporting a TE_{10} mode in terms of refraction at the applicator/tissue interface.

Better approximations to the fields in layered media from rectangular applicators have been reported recently by Bozzetti et al. (1983) and Edenhofer (1983). In these studies coupling between applicator and tissue is taken into account by considering both incident and scattered fields.

Microstrip and Other Compact Applicators

A disadvantage of waveguide applicators is that their dimensions make treatment of some sites (e.g., axilla, neck region) difficult, especially if frequencies below, say, 400 MHz are

Table 1. Characteristics of low-profile applicators

Frequency (MHz)	Material ε	Element size (cm)	Overall dimensions (cm)	Effective penetration depth (cm)	Bolus thickness (cm)
915	30	2.9 diameter	$6 \times 6 \times 1.5$	2.2	1.0
915	10	5×5	$11 \times 11 \times 1.0$	2.4	1.0
430	30	7.8 diameter	$15 \times 25 \times 1.5$	2.8	1.5
200	30	7.5 "D" shaped	$15 \times 25 \times 4.5$	4.0	2.5

used. Another problem is the treatment of large areas on the chest wall where a number of antenna elements on a flexible substrate seem to be useful. To overcome such problems, several workers have developed applicators based on microstrip or similar techniques.

A small ring-type applicator has been described by Bahl et al. (1980), while multielement microstrip applicators have been developed by Tanabe et al. (1983) and Sandhu and Kolozsvary (1984). Since the characteristics of many microstrip applicators depend strongly on the load presented to them, it is important that sufficient bolus is included between the element and tissue to achieve predictable performance from one treatment to another.

Johnson et al. (1984a) have described a series of applicators utilizing some of the microstrip design techniques but which are relatively insensitive to loading conditions. The basic applicator design consists of a thin copper element sandwiched between two slabs of low-loss high-permittivity dielectric material, one of which carries a ground plane. The element is excited by the central conductor of a 50-ohm coaxial cable, the outer of which is connected to the ground plane. The shape of the element may be rectangular or circular or it may be determined empirically with the maximum dimension of the element chosen for resonance in either the $\lambda/2$ or $\lambda/4$ mode.

Table 1 lists some characteristics of these applicators, including the effective penetration depth, measured in muscle phantom, and the thickness of water bolus required to contain near fields associated with the feed points of the elements.

Johnson et al. (1984b) have calculated SAR distributions associated with these compact applicators. Their approximation was to represent the radiating element by two spaced dipoles. The dipoles were treated as 20 adjacent current elements having magnitudes corresponding to a sinusoidal distribution. The electric field at any point in the phantom was computed using ray optics by summing the contributions from each dipole element allowing for loss in the phantom but assuming no loss in the applicator material. Calculations with different spacing and number of dipoles showed that the computed patterns and effective penetration depths were in reasonable agreement with measurements at distances of $\lambda/6$ or more from the radiator with a two-dipole representation. With an applicator of material having $\varepsilon_r = 90$ and muscle phantom, refraction effects were insignificant at 200 MHz. At other frequencies an approximate allowance was made for refraction according to Snell's law.

Some predictions of the model are included in Fig. 7, which shows the dependence of effective penetration depths on frequency for several elements. Experimental data obtained with low-profile applicators are seen to be in good agreement with the model. Some results from Turner and Kumar (1982) for TE_{10} mode waveguide applicators are included for comparison. Their calculations predict little dependence of effective penetra-

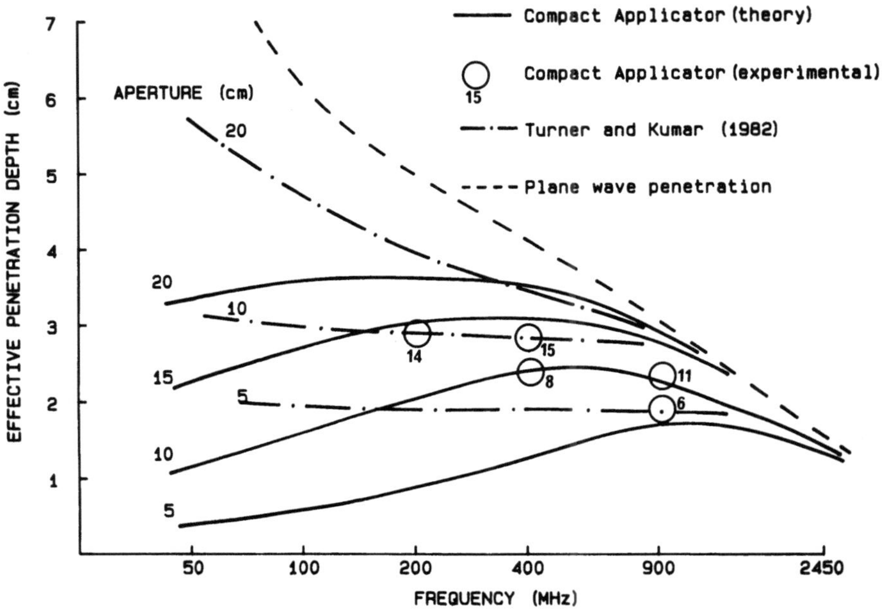

Fig. 7. Dependence of effective penetration depth in plane, semiinfinite muscle medium on frequency and aperture size. (Johnson et al. 1984b)

tion depth on frequency for a given aperture below a particular frequency, behavior which probably arises from the inability of their model to account for diffraction and refraction in the case of apertures which are electrically very small.

Multiple-Applicator Systems

A common limitation in using any single electromagnetic applicator for local heating, especially when tissue curvature is not great, is that the maximum SAR is produced at or near the surface. It follows that, even allowing for skin cooling, adequate temperatures at depths of 3-4 cm are difficult to achieve without producing excessive temperatures in overlying superficial tissues. The use of multiple applicators offers the possibility of field enhancement at depth, while the increased flexibility from controlling the relative phases and amplitudes associated with each applicator is attractive insofar as the shape of heating patterns is modified and the effects of differences in geometry and dielectric and thermal properties are reduced from one tratment to another.

Guerquin-Kern et al. (1980) carried out phantom experiments using two orthogonal applicators and showed that heating at depth was improved when the applicators were driven in phase rather than with a phase difference of 180°. Recently, Nilsson (1984) calculated the absorbed power distribution in a uniform medium due to two waveguide applicators as a function of the relative orientation and phase relationship of the applicators and frequency. The results suggest that significant improvement in the size and uniformity of the heated field may be achieved where this geometry can be used.

The choice of frequency at which a multiple-applicator system operates is based on a compromise between the localization and the penetration required. If heating deep within the human body is required, calculations suggest that a frequency below 100 MHz is necessary (Turner and Kumar 1982; Bach Andersen 1983; Lagendijk 1983), in which case the "focus" is comparable with the dimensions of the body's cross section. Several investigations into the use of higher frequencies, where a localized focus may be produced in more superficial regions, have been reported.

Melek and Anderson (1981) used a ray-tracing technique to study the focussing effects of 17 dipole radiators (2450 MHz) in an elliptic cylindrical phantom. The radiators were arranged in the combinations of semicircular or semielliptical arrays and an orthogonal short linear array and were spaced, in air, from the phantom whose complex permittivity was approximately (22 – j4.3). Their calculations showed that a focus of the order of one wavelength in size and with a global maximum SAR 3 dB greater than the maximum SAR at the surface could be produced at a depth of approximately one plane wave penetration depth (~4.3 cm). However, the phantom represented uniform lung tissue and had significantly lower loss than muscle (attenuation in muscle, ~500 dB/m, cf. attenuation in phantom, 200 dB/m) and so the relatively deep focus reported is unrealistic for cases in which layers of highly attenuating muscle are to be traversed.

Gee et al. (1984) calculated the power deposition in a plane, semi-infinite muscle phantom ($\varepsilon = 47 - j16.2$) due to an array of 2450-MHz horn antennas and showed that a close-packed, hexagonal array of 19 antennas, offset from the tissue by approximately 7λ in high-permittivity material (deionized water), produced a focus with side lobes ~25 dB below the maximum amplitude and a half-power width of approximately one wavelength at a depth of 2.5 cm in muscle. At this depth, the power from a single applicator would be 13 dB below that at the surface.

Arcangeli et al. (1984) reported a rigorous theoretical study of the SAR distribution within a realistic cross section of the human chest due to 50 dielectrically loaded 915-MHz antennas spaced equidistantly around the chest cross section and in close contact with the skin. These calculations pointed to the necessity for phase control of the sources and to the further improvements offered when both phase and amplitude are varied. This study showed a focus with a global maximum SAR in lung tissue, 6–7 cm deep and about a wavelength in linear dimension. This maximum SAR was typically three times that calculated in superficial regions.

A practical limitation in using a multiapplicator array in direct contact with the patient is that the maximum permissible size of each applicator is reduced as the number of applicators is increased. This, in turn, causes a reduction in the effective penetration depth associated with the applicators. For example, the 50 applicators considered in the study by Arcangeli et al. would have apertures with dimensions of approximately 2 cm and consequently an effective penetration depth of about one-half that of plane waves assumed in those calculations.

The relationship between the number of direct-contact applicators and penetration has been discussed by Knoechel (1983) and Johnson et al. (1984b) and implies that applicators must be spaced from the tissues by a low-loss medium if arrays of suitably sized applicators are to be accommodated around the patient.

The studies referred to above suggest that it is feasible that a high-frequency multiapplicator system will produce enhanced-energy deposition within a focus with dimensions of the order of a wavelength at 1–2 penetration depths within tissue. The sensitivity of this focus to the changes in phase and amplitude caused by patient movement, etc. and the performance of real arrays of electrically small applicators have yet to be determined. Finally, the gain in SAR at the focus of such systems is likely to be small and resulting temperature distributions remain to be evaluated.

Conclusions

This paper has discussed field penetration associated with several types of electromagnetic applicator designed for localized hyperthermia.

At frequencies of 10-30 MHz, near-field effects limit effective penetration to 3-4 cm in muscle tissue. At microwave frequencies effective penetration depth depends upon applicator size, tissue geometry, etc. but even at 100-200 MHz it is usually less than 4 cm in muscle tissue.

The use of more than a single applicator offers improvement in field uniformity and size. It is feasible that multiple microwave applicators with phase and amplitude control will produce enhanced-energy deposition within a region with dimensions $\sim\lambda$ at 1-2 penetration depths.

Many aspects of multiple-applicator systems remain to be investigated but the promising results of early studies suggest their development will improve localized heat delivery in clinical hyperthermia.

References

Arcangeli G, Lombardini PP, Lovisolo GA, Marsiglia G, Piatteli M (1984) Focusing of 915 MHz electromagnetic power on deep human tissues: a mathematical model study. IEEE Trans Biomed Eng 31 (1): 47-52

Audet J, Bolomey JC, Pichot C, N'Guyen DD, Chive M, Leroy Y (1980) Electrical characteristics of waveguide applicators for medical applications. J Microwave Power 15 (3): 177-186

Bach Andersen J (1983) Focussing in lossy media. Proceedings URSI Symposium on Electromagnetic Theory, Santiago de Compostela, Spain, August 1983

Bach Andersen J, Baun A, Harmark K, Heinzl L, Raskmark R, Overgaard J (1984) A hyperthermia system using a new type of inductive applicator. IEEE Trans Biomed Eng 31 (1): 21-27

Bahl IJ, Stuchly SS, Stuchly MA (1980) A new microstrip radiator for medical applications. IEEE Trans Microwave Theory Tech 28 (12): 1464-1468

Bozzetti M, De Leo T, Ercoli C (1983) Energy adsorption from waveguides in biological-like media. Alta Freq 52 (3): 185-187

Edenhofer P (1983) Field characteristics of a dual antenna sensor system probing biological tissues. Proceedings URSI Symposium on Electromagnetic Theory, Santiago de Compostela, Spain, August 1983, pp 685-688

Fray C, Khayata N, Papiernik A (1982) TM_{10} admittance and radiation from a flanged open-ended waveguide in layered absorbing media. Arch Elektronik Übertragungstech 36: 107-110

Gee W, Lee S-S, Bong NK, Cain CA, Mittra R, Magin RL (1984) Focused array hyperthermia applicator: theory and experiment. IEEE Trans Biomed Eng 31 (1): 38-46

Guerquin-Kern JL, Palas L, Gautherie M, Fourney-Fayas C, Gimonet E, Prion A, Samsel M (1980) Étude comparative d'applicateurs hyperfréquences (2450 MHz, 434 MHz) sur phantômes et sur pièces opératoires, en vue d'une utilisation thérapeutique de l'hyperthermie microonde en cancérologie. In: Bertaud AJ, Servantie B (eds) Proceedings URSI Symposium Ondes Electromagnétiques et Biologie, Jouy en Josas, July 1980. URSI, CNFRS, Thiais, pp 241-247

Guy AW (1971) Electromagnetic fields and relative heating patterns due to a rectangular aperture source in direct contact with bilayered biological tissue. IEEE Trans Microwave Theory Tech 19 (2): 214-223

Guy AW, Lehmann JF, Stonebridge JB (1974) Therapeutic applications of electromagnetic power. Proc IEEE 62 (1): 55-75

Hand JW, Ledda JL, Evans NTS (1982) Considerations of radiofrequency induction heating for localised hyperthermia. Phys Med Biol 27 (1): 1-16

Harrington RF (1961) Time-harmonic electromagnetic fields. McGraw-Hill, New York

Ho HS (1979) Design of aperture sources for deep heating using electromagnetic energy. Health Phys 37 (6): 743-750

Ho HS, Guy AW, Sigelmann RA, Lehmann JF (1971) Microwave heating of simulated human limbs by aperture sources. IEEE Trans Microwave Theory Tech 19 (2): 224-231

Johnson RH, James JR, Hand JW, Hopewell JW, Dunlop PRC, Dickinson RJ (1984a) New low-profile applicators for local heating of tissues. IEEE Trans Biomed Eng 31 (1): 28-37

Johnson RH, James JR, Hand JW (1984b) Field penetration of multiple compact applicators in localised deep hyperthermia. In: Overgaard J (ed) Hyperthermic oncology, vol 1. Taylor and Francis, London, pp 667-670

Knoechel R (1983) Capabilities of multiapplicator systems for focused hyperthermia. IEEE Trans Microwave Theory Tech 31 (1): 70-73

Lagendijk JJW (1983) A new coaxial TEM radiofrequency/microwave applicator for non-invasive deep-body hyperthermia. J Microwave Power 18 (4): 99-107

Lerch IA, Kohn S (1983) Radiofrequency hyperthermia: the design of coil transducers for local heating. Int J Radiat Oncol Biol Phys 9: 939-948

Melek M, Anderson AP (1981) A thinned cylindrical array for focused microwave hyperthermias. In: Proceedings of the 11th European Microwave Conference. Microwave Exhibitions & Publishers, Tunbridge Wells, pp 427-432

Morita N, Bach Andersen J (1982) Near-field absorption in a circular cylinder from electric and magnetic line sources. Bioelectromagnetics 3: 253-274

Nilsson P (1984) Physics and technique of microwave-induced hyperthermia in the treatment of malignant tumours. Thesis, University of Lund

Robillard M, N'Guyen DD, Chivé M, Leroy Y, Audet J, Bolomey JC, Pichot C (1980) Profondeur de pénétration et résolution spatiale de sondes atraumatiques utilisées en microondes. In: Berteaud AJ, Servantie B (eds) Proceedings URSI Symposium Ondes Electromagnetiques et Biologie, Jouy en Josas, July 1980. URSI, CNFRS, Thiais, pp 213-217

Sandhu TS, Kolozsvary AJ (1984) Conformal hyperthermia applicators. In: Overgaard J (ed) Hyperthermic oncology, vol 1. Taylor and Francis, London, pp 675-678

Tanabe E, McEuen A, Norris CS, Fessenden P, Samulski TV (1983) A multi-element microstrip antenna for local hyperthermia. IEEE MTT-S International Microwave Symposium Digest, pp 183-185

Turner PF, Kumar L (1982) Computer solution for applicator heating pattern. Natl Cancer Inst Monogr 61: 521-523

Wiley JD, Webster JG (1982) Analysis and control of current distribution under circular dispersive electrodes. IEEE Trans Biomed Eng 29 (5): 381-385

The Development of Applicators for Deep-Body Hyperthermia

J. J. W. Lagendijk and A. A. C. de Leeuw

Academisch Ziekenhuis Utrecht, Instituut voor Radiotherapie van de Rijksuniversiteit, Catharijnesingel 101, 3511 CG Utrecht, The Netherlands

Introduction

Controllable heating at depth within the human body is one of the major constraints in the application of hyperthermia in the treatment of deep-seated tumors. Such tumors include tumors of the pancreas, poorly differentiated tumors of the brain, and the higher stages of tumors of the cervix, the stomach, the bladder, and the rectum, which are presently almost untreatable.

The different approaches can be divided into: (1) local deep-body heating, (2) regional deep-body heating, and (3) total-body heating.

Local deep-body heating can be obtained using invasive "interstitial" microwave (Lyons et al. 1984) or resistive (Doss and McCabe 1976; Strohbehn 1983) or ferromagnetic seed implant (Stauffer et al. 1984) techniques. Local noninvasive heating of small tumor volumes using focused ultrasound is under investigation (Fessenden et al. 1984). Total-body hyperthermia is presently undergoing extensive clinical evaluation (van der Zee et al. 1983). Regional deep-body hyperthermia, the heating of whole body areas such as the extremities, the pelvic area, and the thorax, like local heating, is mostly directed to the local tumor process. However, physical limitations of the heating techniques mean that large volumes are heated. Regional deep-body heating is obtained by perfusion techniques (Schraffordt Koops and Oldhoff 1983) or by radiofrequency (RF) heating, which is the subject of this paper.

Several RF heating systems are in a developmental and/or evaluation phase. Mention must be made of the 27-MHz ridged waveguide applicators (Sterzer et al. 1980), the 50- to 110-MHz "annular phased array" of the BSD Corporation (Turner 1982, 1984), the 13.56-MHz "Magnetrode" inductive applicator (Storm et al. 1981), the 13.56-MHz capacitive systems including the Thermotron RF-8 (Hiraoka et al. 1984), the radiative "circumferential gap" applicator (Rasmark and Bach Andersen 1984), and the radiative "coaxial TEM" applicator (Lagendijk 1983).

These RF systems can be divided into capacitive, radiative interference, and inductive techniques. The discussion below will try to give some basic theory with which the potentialities and limitations of these techniques can be judged. Examples of the characteristic absorbed power distributions and of the problems encountered with real patients and some comments on the hardware designs of the practical systems will be given.

Recent Results in Cancer Research. Vol 101

Theory: Homogeneous Tissues

The absorbed power produced by an RF field at point A in tissue is given by:

$$P = \tfrac{1}{2}\,\sigma\,|\mathbf{E}_{A_1}|^2 \qquad (1)$$

with $\mathbf{E}_A$ being the electric field at point A and σ the conductivity of the tissue at point A for the frequency considered. If we use several fields, each producing electric fields $\mathbf{E}_{Ai}$ at point A, the absorbed power at A is given by:

$$P = \tfrac{1}{2}\,\sigma\,\Big|\sum_{i=1}^{i=n} \mathbf{E}_{Ai}\Big|^2 \qquad (2)$$

If, for instance, two fields have the same polarization and strength at point A, the absorbed power intensity can vary from:

$$P = \tfrac{1}{2}\,\sigma\,|\mathbf{E}_{A1} + \mathbf{E}_{A2}|^2 = 0 \qquad (3)$$

if the fields are coherent, but 180° out of phase to:

$$P = \tfrac{1}{2}\,\sigma\,|\mathbf{E}_{A1} + \mathbf{E}_{A2}|^2 = 2\,\sigma\,|\mathbf{E}|^2 \qquad (4)$$

if the fields are coherent and in phase. If the fields are not coherent:

$$P = \tfrac{1}{2}\,\sigma\,|\mathbf{E}_{A_1} + \mathbf{E}_{A_2}|^2 = \sigma\,|\mathbf{E}_{A_1}|^2 + \sigma\,|\mathbf{E}_{A_2}|^2 = \sigma\,|\mathbf{E}_A|^2 \qquad (5)$$

Thus, to determine an absorbed power distribution in a patient heated with a multiple coherent field method, because of the vectorial summation, we must consider not only the absorbed power distribution of each beam but also the phase and polarization relationships between the different fields at each point in the tissue.

According to the equivalence theorem in its primary form proposed by the Dutch physicist Christiaan Huygens (1609–1695), we can simulate the aperture field of an applicator by a large number of electrical dipole sources, each having a polarization, strength, and phase related to the aperture field described (Fig. 1). Increasing the amount of dipole sources increases the accuracy of the solution. The field of each dipole in homogeneous "tissues" is given by the far-field approximation:

$$\mathbf{E}_A = C e^{-j(kr-\Phi)} \sin(\Theta)/|\mathbf{r}| \qquad (6)$$

where Θ is the angle between the distance vector $\mathbf{r}$ and dipole moment $\mathbf{p}$ (Fig. 2), k the complex propagation constant given by $k = k_0\,(\varepsilon' - j\varepsilon'')^{1/2}$, C a constant given the strength

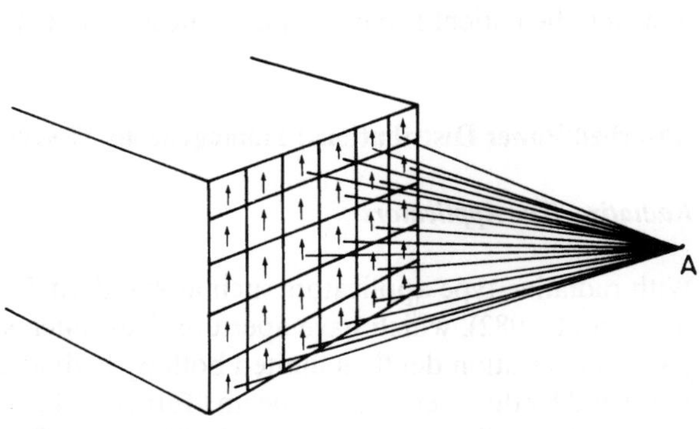

Fig. 1. Aperture field description by dipole simulation. The strength, phase, and polarization of each dipole is given by the part of the aperture field described

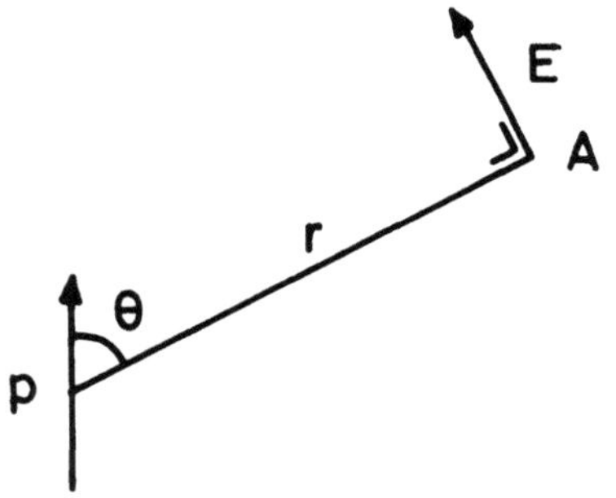

Fig. 2. The radiation field of an electric dipole

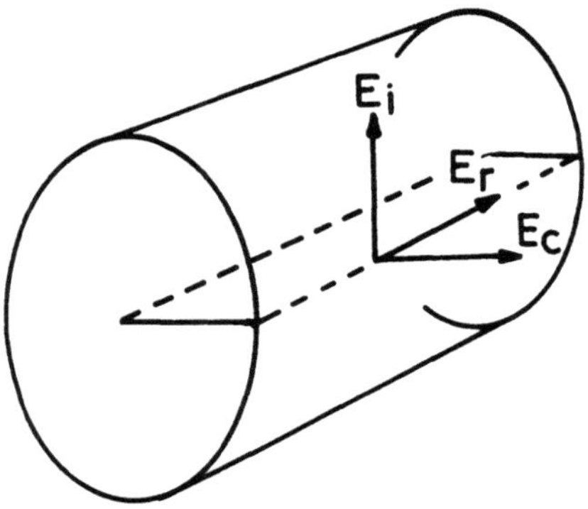

Fig. 3. Orthogonal electric field components at each point of the body surface

of the dipole, Φ the incident phase of the dipole, and ε' and ε'' the dielectric constant and loss factor of the tissue, respectively. **E** is oriented perpendicular to the distance vector **r** in the plane throughout the axis of the dipole. The near-field effects of the dipoles have no physical significance. The real aperture field they describe is uniform in strength over the surface described by each dipole.

Examples of the potential of this description of aperture fields are given by Turner and Kumar (1982), Lagendijk (1983), and Nilsson (1984).

In general, we can describe an RF field by its three orthogonal electric field components at each surface point of the body (Fig. 3). By simulating these fields with dipole sources, we can describe the characteristic absorbed power distributions in homogeneous tissues of the various RF deep-body systems, with the exception of the capacitive system, in which the patient is part of the applicator system.

Absorbed Power Distributions: Homogeneous Tissues

Radiative-Type Applicators

With radiative-type applicators such as standard TE_{10} waveguide or stripline applicators (Bahl et al. 1982), which have aperture sizes much smaller than body diameter, the half-power penetration depth is limited both by high attenuation of tissue (Johnson and Guy 1972) and by divergence of the beam (Turner and Kumar 1982). Even with 27-MHz ridged waveguide applicators (Sterzer et al. 1980), the effective half-power penetration depth is less than 2.1 cm when a single applicator is used (van Rhoon et al. 1984).

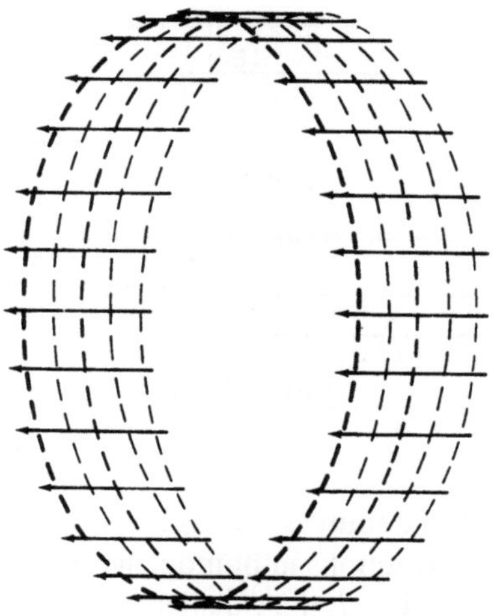

Fig. 4. Ideal uniform circumferential electric field distribution for optimal radiative deep-body heating. The patient must be positioned inside the ring with the area to be heated in the plane through the center of the ring. *Broken lines,* H-field; *arrows,* E-field

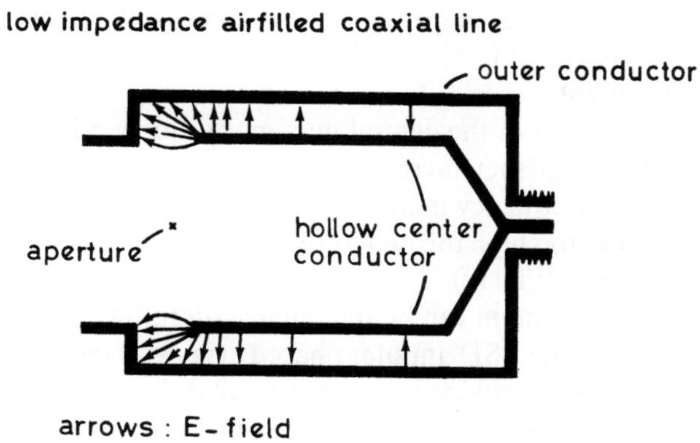

Fig. 5. Cross-section of "coaxial TEM" applicator (operating principle)

To produce sufficient deep-body heating, it is necessary to have constructive interference among several small applicators or one applicator that produces an aperture field of such a kind that constructive interference occurs. These applicator systems or applicators are characterized by a more or less uniform circumferential electric field (Fig. 4) with orientation $\mathbf{E}_r$ (Fig. 3), which is limited to a well-defined aperture. An example of the multiple applicator approach is the BSD (Turner 1982, 1984) annular phased array system. With this system, the circumferential **E**-field is made by 16 small applicators, which are divided into two rings of 8 applicators each, together making an aperture with a width of 46 cm. The "circumferential gap" applicator (Rasmark and Bach Andersen 1984) and the coaxial TEM applicator (Lagendijk 1983) produce uniform circumferential E-fields, and with both of them the aperture widths can be varied.

With the coaxial TEM applicator, the aperture field is made by modifying the field of a coaxial line with large inner and outer diameter (Fig. 5). As with the BSD annular phased array (Gibbs et al. 1984), the patient is matched to the aperture by a distilled water bolus (Fig. 6). Because of its coaxial structure, the applicator is not limited in frequency bandwidth.

The deep-body heating capabilities of these systems depend on the operating frequency and the width of the aperture. If we simulate the radiating aperture with a large number of

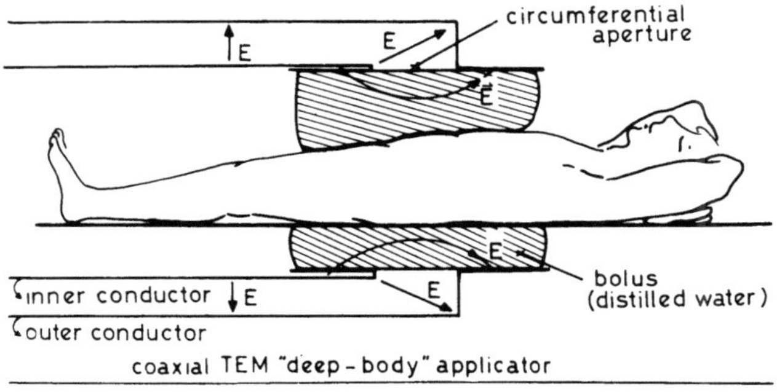

Fig. 6. Prototype design clinical "coaxial TEM" applicator system

dipole sources, as has been described, we can calculate the characteristic absorbed power distributions in homogeneous "tissues."

In Fig. 7, the calculated absorbed power distribution is given for a cylindrical phantom 30 cm in diameter, which is heated with 70 MHz. The aperture width is 24 cm.

Broadening the aperture width improves the intensity of the central maximum. However, with increasing aperture width the axial length of the absorbed power distribution also increases (Fig. 8), which intensifies the problems associated with systemic heating of the patient.

The width of the central maximum is dependent on the wavelength in tissue. Decreasing the frequency increases the radial width of the maximum (Fig. 9).

If the frequency increases the radial width becomes narrow. However, if the frequency becomes too high the penetration obtained is not enough to produce a central interference maximum (Fig. 10).

The maximum can be steered by controlling the phase of segments of the aperture field (Fig. 11). The BSD annular phased array and the circumferential gap applicator are potentially able to provide this steering capability, whereas the coaxial TEM applicator, with its present single coaxial feeding point, provides only limited steering capabilities. With steering techniques, problems must be expected due to cross-coupling between applicator segments or applicator pairs, which produce difficulties in matching the power generators to the applicator segments or applicators.

Inductive-Type Applicators

Most inductive-type deep-body hyperthermia systems have a concentric coil (Oleson 1984). We can describe the field of the coil by replacing the wire with a large amount of dipole sources oriented along E_i (Figs. 3, 12). Phase and strength remain the same provided that the wire length of the coil is small in comparison with the wavelength. The characteristic absorbed power distribution (Fig. 13) is independent of the frequency, as long as the body diameter is small in comparison with the plane wave half-power penetration depth and with the wavelength in the tissue. The central minimum occurs by destructive interference of the dipole fields.

Remarkable effects occur when the frequency increases and the penetration depth decreases. For a single-turn 27-MHz coil, assuming a constant phase over the coil, the power maximum shifts from the skin toward deeper layers. The tissue wavelength, which is no longer great in comparison with the body diameter, causes phase rotation along the distance vector **r** from each dipole to the point A in the tissue considered. This phase rota-

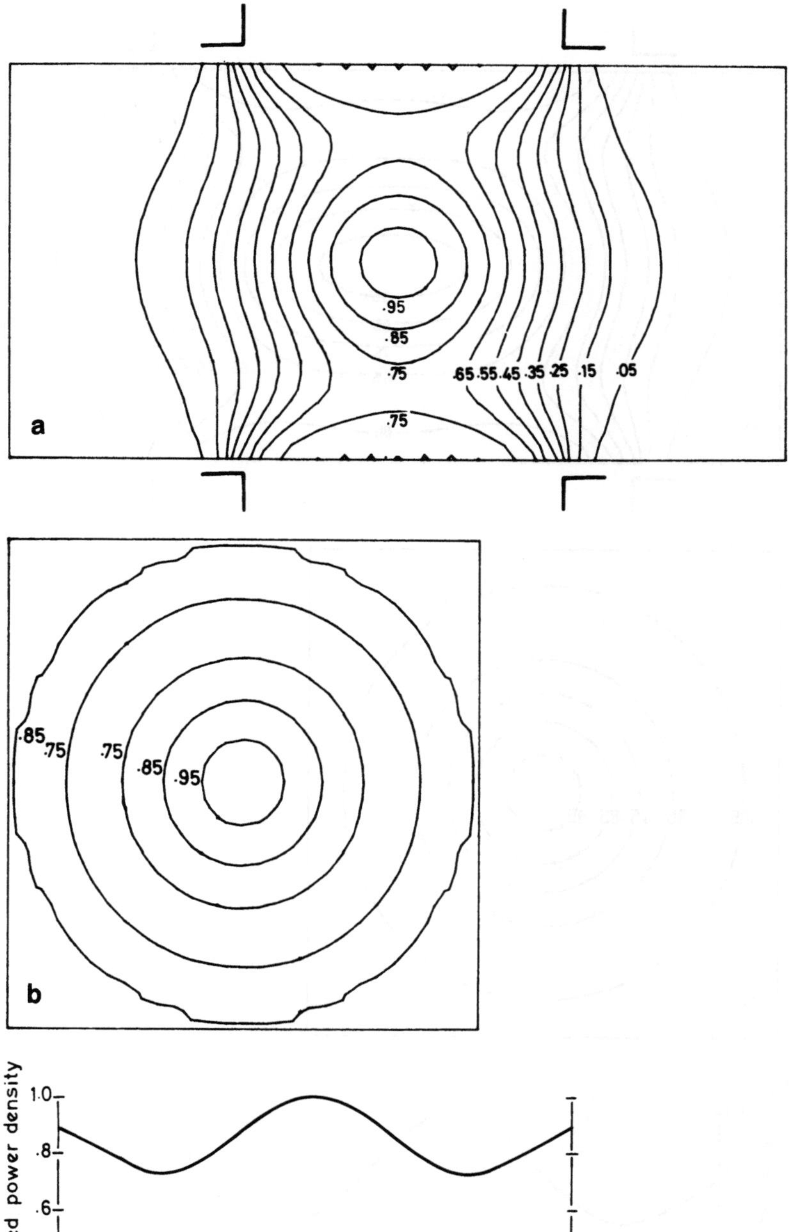

Fig. 7 a–c. Calculated three-dimensional absorbed power distribution for a 30-cm diameter homogeneous phantom heated with a "coaxial TEM" applicator. Frequency, 70 MHz; phantom properties, $\varepsilon^* = 80 - j210$; aperture width, 24 cm (simulated by 13 rings of 32 dipoles). Distributions are normalized to central maximum. **a** axial distribution; **b** radial distribution; **c** distribution along line through the center of the radial aperture plane

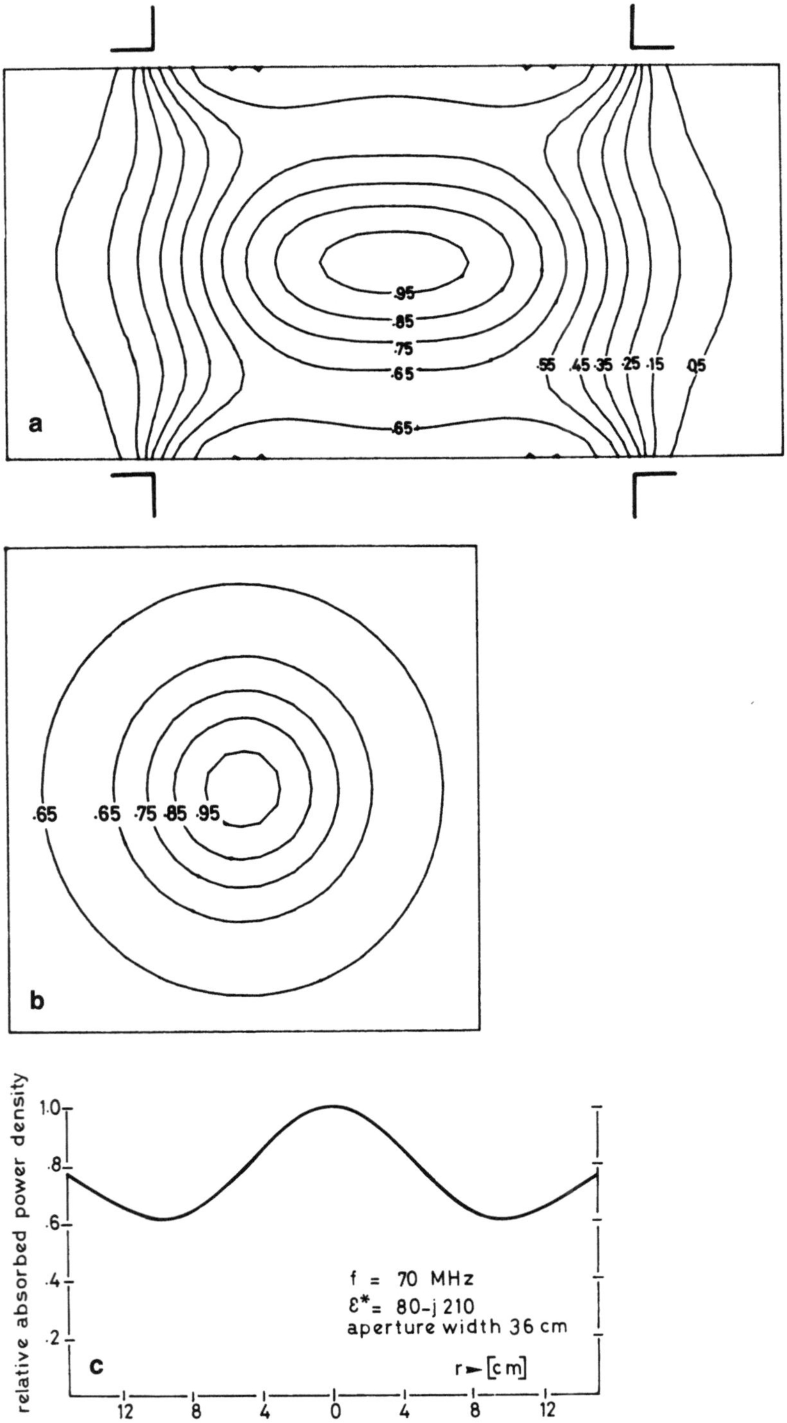

Fig. 8a–c. Situation of Fig. 7 now with an aperture width of 36 cm

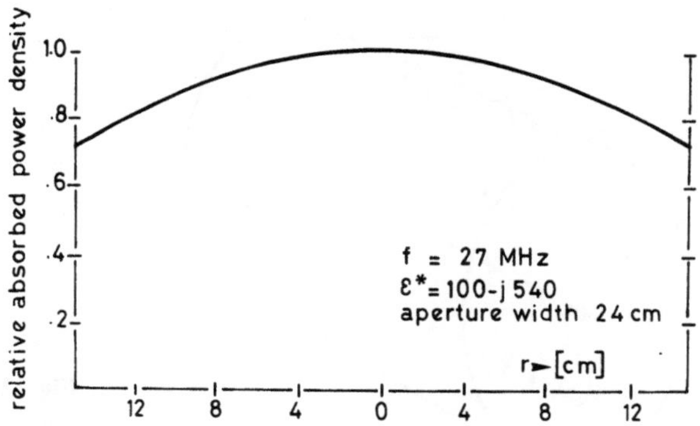

Fig. 9. Situation of Fig. 7 now with 27 MHz and phantom properties $\varepsilon^* = 100 - j540$. Only the distribution along a line through the center of the radial aperture plane is given

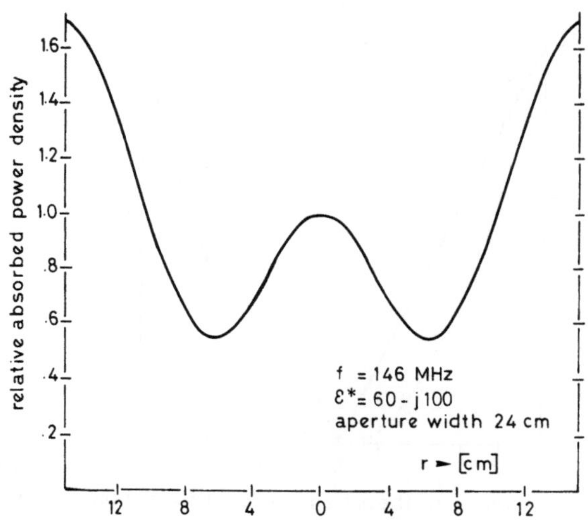

Fig. 10. Situation of Fig. 7 now with 146 MHz and phantom properties $\varepsilon^* = 60 - j100$. Only the distribution along a line through the center of the radial aperture plane is given

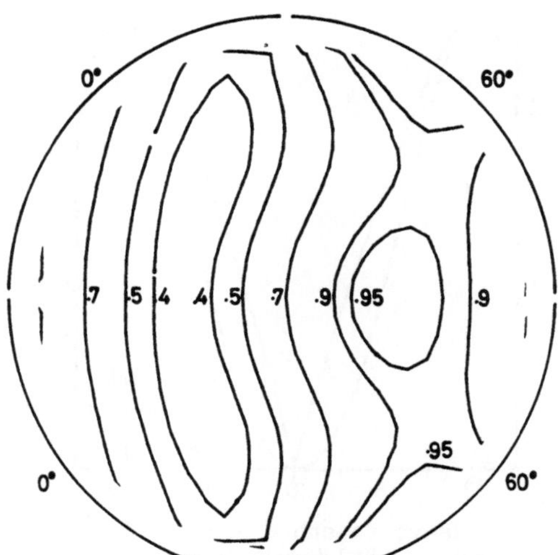

Fig. 11. Steering of central maximum by phase shifting of parts of the aperture field. Situation of Fig. 7 with the applicator divided into four segments with phase respectively 0°, 0°, 60°, and 60°, all segments equal intensity

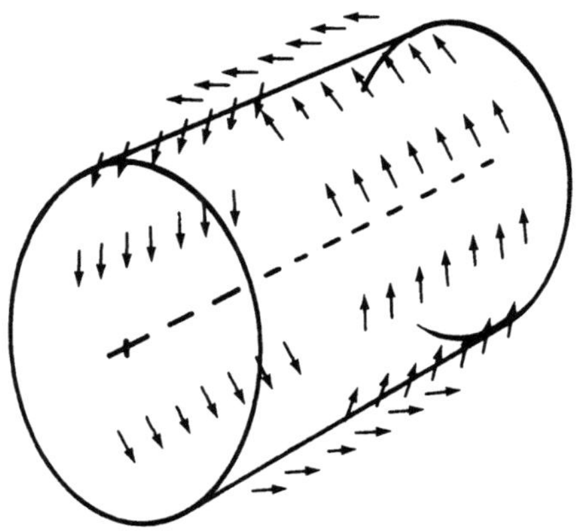

Fig. 12. Electric dipole simulation of inductive concentric coil applicator system. *Arrows*, dipole sources

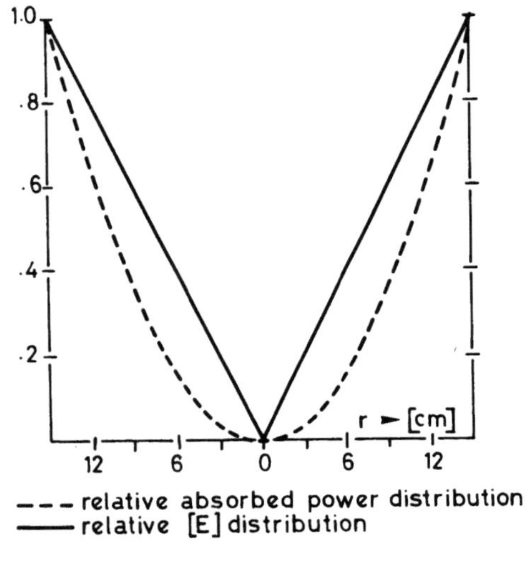

Fig. 13. Specific **E**-field and absorbed power distribution of inductive concentric coil applicator operating on low frequencies. Phantom diameter, 30 cm

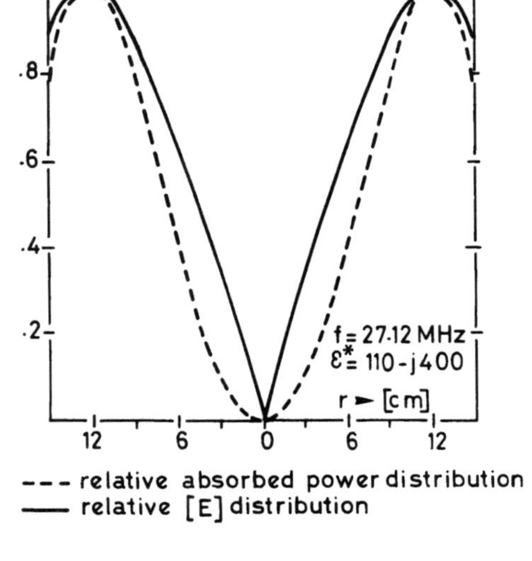

Fig. 14. E-field and absorbed power distribution at 27 MHz; phantom properties, $\varepsilon^* = 110 - j400$; phantom diameter, 30 cm

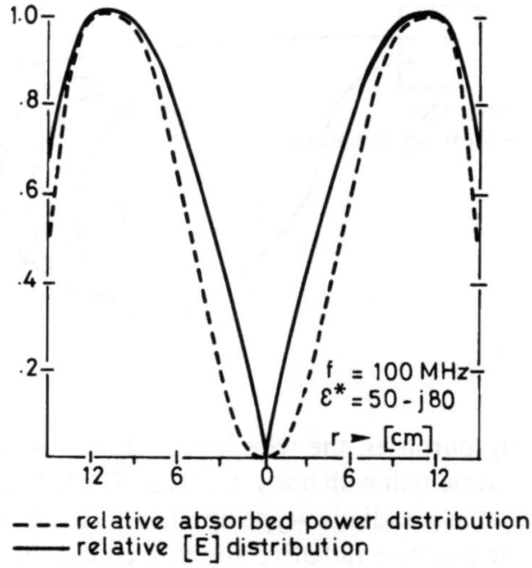

Fig. 15. E-field and absorbed power distribution of inductive coil at 100 MHz. Phantom properties, $\varepsilon^* = 50 - j80$; phantom diameter, 30 cm

tion, together with the decreasing penetration depth at higher frequencies, results in a decreasing destructive interference. If frequency increases further, constructive interference occurs (Fig. 14). If the tissue wavelength is equal to the body diameter, for example, constructive interference occurs halfway between the body surface and the central body axis (Fig. 15). However, at these high frequencies, there is phase rotation over the coil wire, which disturbs the ideal situation. This wire-phase rotation must be taken into consideration when calculating the absorbed power distributions of these high-frequency coils.

Because of the central minimum, which is essential for all inductive systems, these techniques are of no use for real deep-body hyperthermia.

Planar coils and coaxial pairs of coils (Oleson 1984) give doughnut-shaped absorbed power distributions, which are unusable for deep-body heating, as can be calculated with the theory described.

Capacitive-Type Systems

For capacitive systems, which are characterized by an **E**-field polarization oriented as $\mathbf{E}_c$ (Fig. 3), the situation is different. With these systems, as with the resistive systems [local current field systems (Doss and McCabe 1976)], the patient's body is a direct part of the applicator system. For wavelengths that are large in comparison with body diameter, the absorbed power distribution can be calculated using a quasi-static solution of the electric field potential (Doss 1982; Wiley and Webster 1982). These calculations show rapid field decay away from the surface if the plates are small in comparison with the distance between the plates and rather uniform if the plates are large in proportion to the distance between them.

Helical Coil Systems

With helical coil systems (Fig. 16) such as have been described by Ruggera and Kantor (1984), the wire of the coil is about as long as the wavelength. This implies a phase shift along the coil which produces an axial electric field oriented along $\mathbf{E}_r$ (Fig. 3). For match-

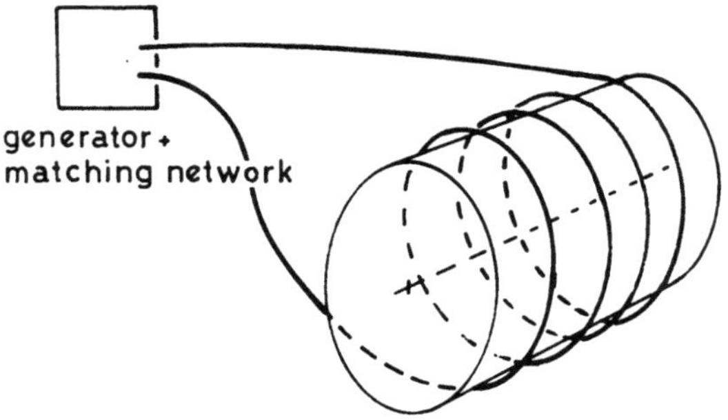

Fig. 16. Helical coil applicator configuration

ing purposes, the wire length chosen is mostly one-half or one whole wavelength (wire wavelength with body in place). The helical coil acts both as an inductive applicator (p. 22) and as a radiative-type applicator (p. 20). With the one-half wavelength coil, for instance, the effective radiative aperture equals the axial length of the coil. Because of the low operating frequency (13.56 or 27.12 MHz), the radiative part of the absorbed power distribution is uniform across the diameter of the body (Fig. 10). The inductive component is almost negligible because of the low coupling efficiency of the inductive **E**-field component. The inductive coupling is much lower than the radiative one, which is due to destructive interference of the inductive **E**-field. The exact three-dimensional absorbed power distribution can be calculated using the dipole description of the coil field. Because a water bolus cannot be used to match the coil to the patient, the axial length of the coil is small in comparison with the wavelength in the air surrounding the coil, thus producing a bad impedance match, an absorbed power distribution of great axial length, and a large stray field.

Theory: Inhomogeneous Phantoms

The calculation of the absorbed power distribution in homogeneous tissues gave us a clue as to the specific heating potentialities of the various deep-body applicators.

Because of the great variety of complex dielectric constants in the human body, we need a better solution of the absorbed power distributions to judge and optimize the different heating systems. Real three-dimensional calculation of the absorbed power distributions is hindered by the limitations of present-day computer systems (van den Berg et al. 1983; Iskander et al. 1982) and by the limited anatomical data available for each individual patient. Modern 16- and 32-bit large-memory personal computers will help solve the computer problem within a few years. A program for two-dimensional absorbed power calculations is already available for a large-memory IBM-PC computer (van den Berg, personal communication). Anatomical data, especially of soft tissue structures, is becoming available with the advent of nuclear magnetic resonance (NMR) imaging (Bakker and Vriend 1984).

To evaluate the present heating systems and the value of the two-dimensional computational models, the basic inhomogeneity, an interface between two different tissues, must be considered. Across a tissue interface, for which the complex dielectric constant changes discontinuously, the tangential components of the electric field **E** and the magnetic field **H** must be continuous. This also means the continuity of the normal components of the electrical ($D_n = \varepsilon E_n$) and magnetic ($B_n = \mu H_n$) flux density.

Table 1. Ratios between the absorbed power intensities in fat and muscle for **E** parallel to the fat (bone)-muscle tissue interface and **E** normal to the tissue interface. Dielectric constants are according to Johnson and Guy (1972)

Frequency	Dielectric constant		P_f/P_m Parallel	P_f/P_m Normal
	Fat	Muscle		
27.12	20 −j10.2	113−j400	0.025	8.7
40.68	14.6−j 7.9	97−j302	0.026	9.5
100	7.5−j 4.5	72−j159	0.028	11.3
200	6.0−j 3.1	57−j 90	0.034	8.6
300	5.7−j 2.4	54−j 69	0.035	7.0
434	5.6−j 2.0	53−j 49	0.041	6.1
915	5.6−j 1.4	51−j 25	0.056	5.4
2450	5.5−j 0.8	47−j 16	0.052	4.1

To explain the importance of these boundary conditions, we shall consider a fat-muscle interface at 100 MHz. The complex dielectric constant of fat is given by: 7.43−j4.5 ($\sigma_f = 0.025$ mho/m), that of muscle by: 71.7−j159 ($\sigma_m = 0.889$ mho/m) (Johnson and Guy 1972). For the situation in which the entire **E**-field is parallel to the tissue interface ($\mathbf{E}_n = 0$), we find a ratio between the absorbed power in fat and muscle of:

$$\left.\begin{array}{l}\dfrac{P_f}{P_m} = \dfrac{\sigma_f|\mathbf{E}_f|^2}{\sigma_m|\mathbf{E}_m|^2} \\ \mathbf{E}_f = \mathbf{E}_m\end{array}\right\} \quad \frac{P_f}{P_m} = \frac{\sigma_f}{\sigma_m} = 0.028 \tag{7}$$

For the situation in which the entire **E**-field is perpendicular to the tissue interface we find:

$$\left.\begin{array}{l}\dfrac{P_f}{P_m} = \dfrac{\sigma_f|\mathbf{E}_f|^2}{\sigma_m|\mathbf{E}_m|^2} \\ \varepsilon_f^*\mathbf{E}_f = \varepsilon_m^*\mathbf{E}_m\end{array}\right\} \quad \frac{P_f}{P_m} = \frac{\sigma_f}{\sigma_m} \cdot \frac{|\varepsilon_m^*|^2}{|\varepsilon_f^*|^2} = 11.3 \tag{8}$$

Table 1 gives the ratios between the absorbed power intensities in fat and muscle, depending on the orientation of the **E**-field for several frequencies. The dielectric constants are according to Johnson and Guy (1972).

These considerable differences in absorbed power in fat and muscle, depending solely on the field orientation, are of extreme importance in understanding the problems of RF deep-body heating. The reflected waves generated by these boundary conditions produce interference patterns inside the tissue structures, provided that the wavelength in tissue is not large compared with these structures.

Absorbed Power Distributions: Structured Tissues

Capacitive-Type Systems

With capacitive heating the electric field is perpendicular to the subcutaneous fat-muscle interface, which results in extreme heating of fat, as shown in Table 1. If the layer of fat is thin, cooling of the skin by the relatively cold underlying muscles can prevent overheating. Hiraoka et al. (1984) showed that when the thickness of the subcutaneous fat was greater than 2 cm, efficient deep-body hyperthermia was limited by fat heating in 48% of their patients. Calculations made by Armitage et al. (1983) of the absorbed power distribution produced by capacitive heating of the thoracic region show inhomogeneous distributions caused by tissue structures and field divergence, with heating concentrated mostly in the thoracic wall structures.

Radiative-Type Systems

Calculations of the absorbed power distributions produced by radiative systems in structured tissues have been presented, among others, by van den Berg et al. (1983) and Iskander et al. (1982). Their calculations are essentially two dimensional, with the result that their **E**-field is always oriented parallel to the body axis and the tissue interfaces. This results in fat and bone heating that is minimal compared with the absorbed power intensity in organs, muscles, and tumor. With real radiative heating systems, we do have axial **E**-field orientation in the central plane through the aperture, but the actual absorbed power distribution is more complex than predicted with the two-dimensional models. We can distinguish between two complicating factors:

1. The bending of the **E**-field if we look at locations outside the central plane (Fig. 17), producing **E**-fields perpendicular to the main muscle-subcutaneous fat interface
2. The existence of complex tissue interfaces that are more or less perpendicular to the body axis (Fig. 18)

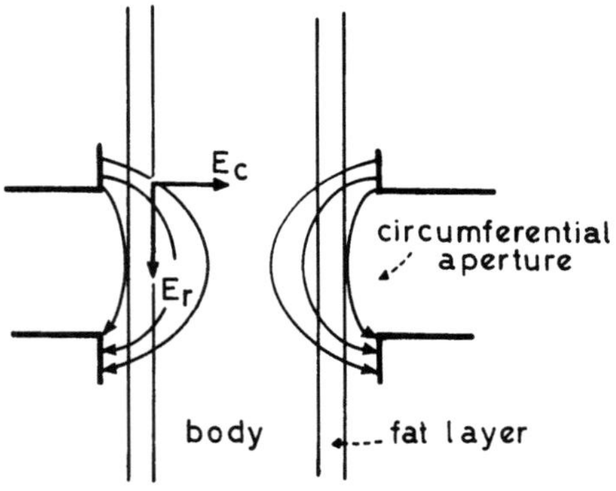

Fig. 17. **E**-fields perpendicular to muscle-subcutaneous fat interfaces due to limited aperture width

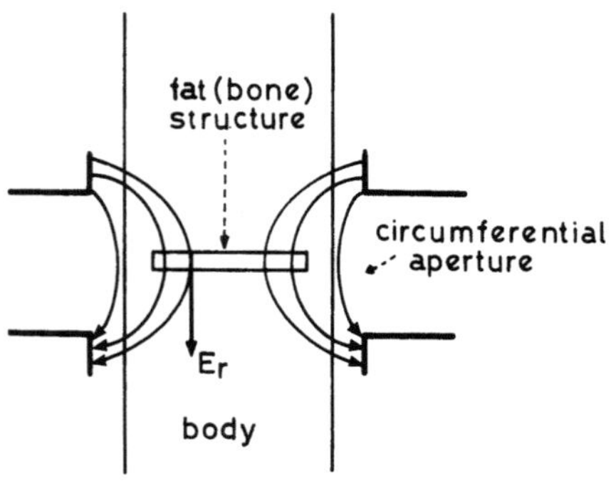

Fig. 18. **E**-fields normal to tissue interfaces by tissue anatomy

These complicating factors can produce severe problems because of the high fat and bone absorption related to them (Table 1). Figures 19–21 show some examples of the absorbed power distribution in structured phantoms generated with a 20-cm-diameter coaxial TEM applicator (Lagendijk 1983) and operating for experimental simplicity at 434 MHz on a scaled phantom. Preferential fat (bone) heating occurs with these geometries. Figure 19a gives the experimental situation. The conductivity of the high water content "muscle" phantom (Guy 1971) has been decreased by lowering the salt content (0.3% saline solution). The fat phantom has a dielectric constant $\varepsilon^* = 6.7 - j1.3$, a density of 1.2 g/cm^3, and a specific heat of 2.04 Jg^{-1} K^{-1}. Figure 19b gives the thermographic image of the temperature distribution after a 2.5-min microwave power pulse of 130 W. The temperature of the fat (bone) layer has been lowered by heat conduction during the power pulse and the 1-min measurement time. Measurements of the absorbed power density in the central phantom region obtained with a Luxtron nondisturbing temperature measurement system using short power pulse techniques give a ratio between fat and muscle for absorbed power density of $P_f/P_m = 5$. Figure 20a gives a similar experimental situation, with Fig. 20b showing both boundary conditions described: the high "muscle" absorption at the boundary parallel to the **E**-field and the absorbed power minimum in muscle at the boundary perpendicular to the **E**-field. Figure 21a gives the experimental simulation of the pelvic bone structures, in this case with a muscle phantom according to Guy (1971) but prepared with a 0.6% saline solution. Figure 21b shows the preferential heating of the bone structures and the field distribution in the muscle tissue. Local pain in the upper thigh, as described by Emami et al. (1984) using the annular phased array, can be caused by this phenomenon owing to preferential heating of the pelvic bone structures.

If the distance between the aperture and the body surface is small, as with the circumferential gap applicator (Raskmark and Bach Andersen 1984), or if the aperture width and water bolus are small, heating in subcutaneous fat layers can be expected (Fig. 17) with extreme **E**-field bending perpendicular to the tissue interfaces.

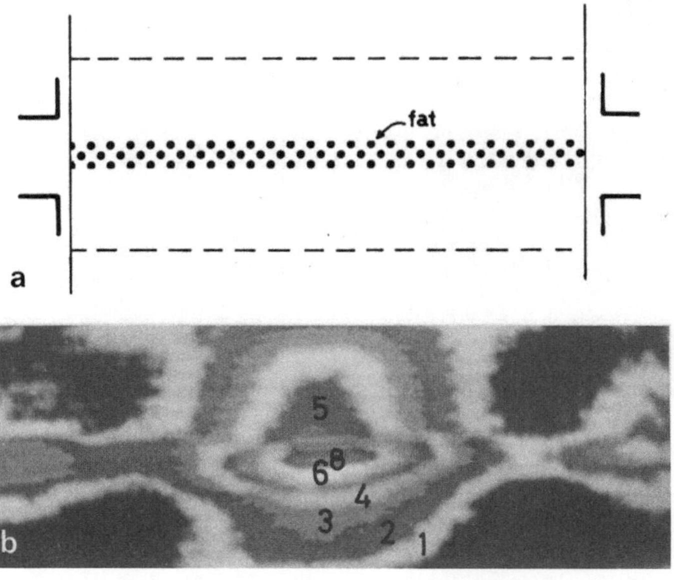

Fig. 19. a Experimental situation. Structured phantom heated with a 20-cm-diameter "coaxial TEM" applicator. **b** Thermographic image of temperature distribution after a 2.5-min microwave pulse of 130 W. Temperature difference between isotherms is 0.45 °C

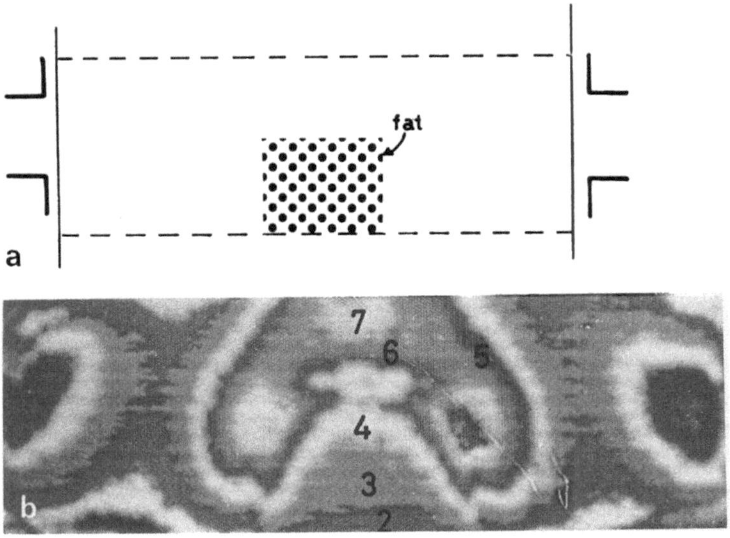

Fig. 20. **a** Experimental situation. Structured phantom heated with a 20-min-diameter "coaxial TEM" applicator. **b** Thermographic image of temperature distribution after a 4.0-min microwave pulse of 130 W. Temperature difference between isotherms is 0.40 °C

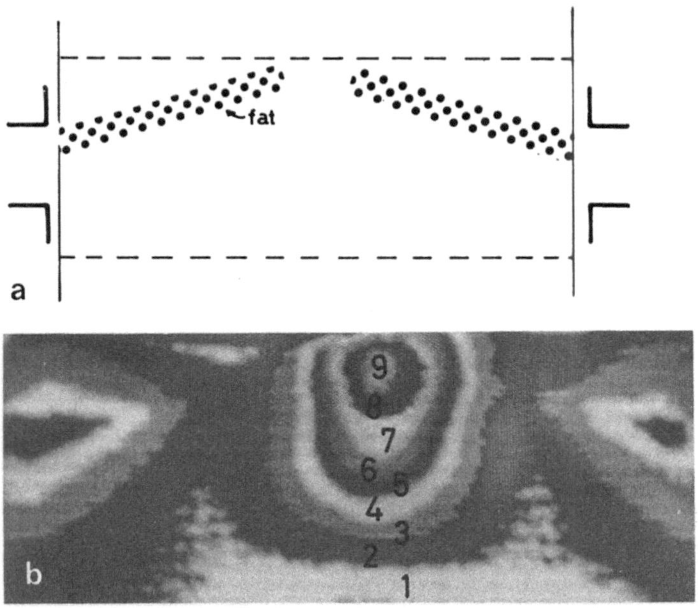

Fig. 21. **a** Experimental situation. Structured phantom heated with a 20-cm-diameter "coaxial TEM" applicator. **b** Thermographic image of temperature distribution after a 5.0-min microwave pulse of 130 W. Temperature difference between isotherms is 0.90 °C

Inductive-Type Systems

Only superficial structures can be heated with inductive heating systems (Fig. 13). Since the **E**-field is parallel to the main subcutaneous fat-muscle interfaces, fat absorption is low. However, tissue interfaces perpendicular to the **E**-field, such as bone structures, can still produce inhomogeneous heating. Armitage et al. (1983) also calculated the inductive deep-body hyperthermia systems, which confirm the existence of the central minimum and the inhomogeneous absorption in the superficial regions.

Helical Coil Systems

The helical coil systems have the advantages and disadvantages of radiative-type systems because they have a nonuseful inductive field component. The absorbed power distributions of helical coils in structured phantoms can be evaluated by a separate look at the two field components.

Conclusions

The characteristic absorbed power distributions in homogeneous tissues of inductive and radiative systems can be evaluated by dipole simulation of the electric field aperture. Capacitive systems require a quasi-static solution of the electric field potential.

The capacitive systems are limited by subcutaneous fat heating and low effective penetration depth. Inductive systems are characterized by an absolute central power minimum. Inductive concentric coil systems operating at higher frequencies need special attention. If destructive interference is decreased it seems that reasonable regional heating of tissues situated off the central axis will be feasible. However, because of the doughnut-shaped absorbed power distribution, large tissue volumes are heated unnecessarily. Radiative systems offer the best deep-body heating capabilities and provide more or less useful absorbed power distributions, especially at frequencies round 70 MHz. The absorbed power maximum produced can be steered through the body; however, because of the rather uniform heating throughout the whole-body cross section, the heating essentially remains regional. Careful attention must be given to the fundamental preferential heating of fat and bone structures with tissue interfaces perpendicular to the **E**-field, which can limit the potential for clinical application of radiative deep-body heating systems. This preferential heating of "low-loss" structures, related to **E**-field orientation, also occurs at high-frequency microwave heating. Heating head and neck tumors using 434- or 915-MHz microwave techniques, for example, can cause severe overheating of the jaw bones when the **E**-field polarization is perpendicular to these bones.

Finally, taking into account the fundamental inhomogeneities in temperature distribution caused by the local cooling of large blood vessels (Lagendijk 1982; Lagendijk and Mooibroek, this volume) and the limitations of invasive thermometry (Hand 1984), we can conclude that the laws of physics are not with us in the application of hyperthermia.

References

Armitage DW, LeVeen HH, Pethig R (1983) Radiofrequency-induced hyperthermia: computer simulation of specific absorption rate distributions using realistic anatomical models. Phys Med Biol 28 (1): 31-42

Bahl IJ, Stuchly SS, Lagendijk JJW, Stuchly MA (1982) Microstrip loop radiators for medical applications. IEEE Trans Microwave Theory Tech 30 (7): 1090-1093

Bakker CJG, Vriend J (1984) Multi-exponential water proton spin-lattice relaxation in biological tissues and its implications for quantitative NMR-imaging. Phys Med Biol 29 (5): 509-518

Doss JD (1982) Calculation of electric fields in conductive media. Med Phys 9 (4): 566-573

Doss JD, McCabe CW (1976) A technique for localized heating in tissue: an adjunct to tumor therapy. Med Instrum 10 (1): 16-21

Emami B, Perez C, Nussbaum G, Leybovich L (1984) Regional hyperthermia in treatment of recurrent deep-seated tumors: preliminary report. In: Overgaard J (ed) Hyperthermic oncology, vol 1. Taylor and Francis, London, pp 605-608 (Summary papers)

Fessenden P, Lee ER, Anderson TL, Strohbehn JW, Meyer JL, Samulski TV, Marmor JB (1984) Experience with a multitransducer ultrasound system for localized hyperthermia of deep tissues. IEEE Trans Biomed Eng 31: 126-135

Gibbs FA, Sapozink MD, Gates KS, Stewart JR (1984) Regional hyperthermia with an Annular Phased Array in the experimental treatment of cancer: report of work in progress with technical emphasis. IEEE Trans Biomed Eng 31: 115-119

Guy AW (1971) Analyses of electromagnetic fields induced in biological tissues by thermographic studies on equivalent phantom models. IEEE Trans Microwave Theory Tech 19 (2): 205-214

Hand JW (1985) Thermometry in hyperthermia. In: Overgaard J (ed) Hyperthermic oncology, vol 2. Taylor a. Francis, London, pp 299-308

Hiraoka M, Jo S, Takahashi M, Abe M (1984) Thermometry results of RF capacitive heating for human deep-seated tumors. In: Overgaard J (ed) Hyperthermic oncology, vol 1. Taylor and Francis, London, pp 609-612 (Summary papers)

Iskander MF, Turner PF, DuBow JB, Kao J (1982) Two-dimensional technique to calculate the EM power deposition patterns in the human body. J Microwave Power 17: 175-185

Johnson CC, Guy AW (1972) Nonionizing electromagnetic wave effects in biological materials and systems. Proc IEEE 60 (6): 692-718

Lagendijk JJW (1982) The influence of blood flow in large vessels on the temperature distribution in hyperthermia. Phys Med Biol 27: 17-23

Lagendijk JJW (1983) A new coaxial TEM radiofrequency/microwave applicator for non-invasive deep-body hyperthermia. J Microwave Power 18: 367-376

Lyons BE, Britt RH, Strohbehn JW (1984) Localized hyperthermia in the treatment of malignant brain tumours using an interstitial microwave antenna array. IEEE Trans Biomed Eng 31: 53-62

Nilsson P (1984) Physics and techniques of microwave induced hyperthermia in the treatment of malignant tumours. Thesis, University of Lund

Oleson J (1984) A review of magnetic induction methods for hyperthermic treatment of cancer. IEEE Trans Biomed Eng 31: 91-97

Rasmark P, Bach Andersen J (1984) Electronically steered heating of a cylinder. In: Overgaard J (ed) Hyperthermic oncology, vol 1. Taylor and Francis, London, pp 617-620 (Summary papers)

Ruggera P, Kantor G (1984) Development of a family of RF helical coil applicators which produce transversally uniform axially distributed heating in cylindrical fat-muscle phantoms. IEEE Trans Biomed Eng 31: 98-105

Schraffordt Koops H, Oldhoff J (1983) Hyperthermic regional perfusion in high-risk stage-I malignant melanomas of the extremities. Recent Results Cancer Res 86: 223-228

Stauffer PR, Cetas TC, Jones RC (1984) Magnetic induction heating of ferromagnetic implants for inducing localized hyperthermia in deep-seated tumors. IEEE Trans Biomed Eng 31: 235-251

Sterzer F, Paglione RW, Mendecki J, Botstein C (1980) RF therapy for malignancy. IEEE Spectrum 1980 Dec: 32-37

Storm FK, Harrison WH, Elliot RS, Kaiser LR, Silberman AW, Morton DL (1981) Clinical radiofrequency hyperthermia by magnetic-loop induction. J Microwave Power 16 (2): 179-184

Strohbehn JW (1983) Temperature distributions from interstitial RF electrode hyperthermia systems: theoretical predictions. Int J Radiat Oncol Biol Phys 9: 1655-1667

Turner PF (1982) Deep heating of cylindrical or elliptical masses. J Natl Cancer Inst Monogr 61: 493-495

Turner PF (1984) Regional hyperthermia with an annular phased array. IEEE Trans Biomed Eng 31: 106-114

Turner PF, Kumar L (1982) Computer solution for applicator heating patterns. J Natl Cancer Inst Monogr 61: 521-523

Van den Berg PM, de Hoop AT, Segal A, Praagman N (1983) A computational model of the electromagnetic heating of biological tissue with application to hyperthermic cancer therapy. IEEE Trans Biomed Eng 30 (2): 797-805

Van der Zee J, van Rhoon GC, Wike Hooley JL, Faithfull NS, Reinhold HS (1983) Whole-body hyperthermia in cancer therapy: a report of a phase I-II study. Eur J Cancer Clin Oncol 19 (9): 1189-1200

Van Rhoon GC, Visser AG, van den Berg PM, Reinhold HS (1984) Temperature depth profiles obtained in muscle-equivalent phantoms using the RCA 27 MHz ridged waveguide. In: Overgaard J (ed) Hyperthermic oncology, vol 1. Taylor and Francis, London, pp 499-502

Wiley JD, Webster JG (1982) Analysis and control of the current distribution under circular dispersive electrodes. IEEE Trans Biomed Eng 29: 391-395

Heating of a Rhabdomyosarcoma of the Rat by 2450 MHz Microwaves: Technical Aspects and Temperature Distributions

F. Zywietz, R. Knöchel, and J. Kordts

Universitäts-Krankenhaus Eppendorf, Institut für Biophysik und Strahlenbiologie, Martinistrasse 52, 2000 Hamburg 20, FRG

Introduction

A variety of radiobiological and clinical results have clearly established the therapeutic potential of hyperthermia in cancer treatment, either alone or in combination with other modes of treatment such as ionizing radiation or chemotherapy cf. reviews (Bicher and Bruley 1982; Christensen and Durney 1981; Dewey and Freeman 1980; Field and Bleehen 1979; Gauthérie and Albert 1982; Hahn 1982; Jain and Gullino 1980; Oleson and Dewhirst 1983; Storm 1983) and recent symposia (Dethlefsen 1982; Field and Streffer 1982; Hill 1982; Milder 1979; Overgaard 1984; Streffer and van Beuningen 1963). Several methods are presently being investigated for heat production; however, for localized hyperthermia treatment radiowaves, microwaves, and ultrasound are widely used. (Cheung 1982; Guy and Chen 1983; Hand and ter Haar 1981; Hunt 1982). These methods have the advantage of being noninvasive to the tumor, except temperature monitoring and interstitial techniques.

In a previous study, the effect of microwave heating on the radiation response of the rhabdomyosarcoma of the rat was investigated by heating the tumors with a manually controlled microwave device (Zywietz 1982). Manual control of hyperthermia was found to be both tedious and, to some extent, inaccurate. If larger groups of tumors are to be treated some form of automatic heating system is desirable. At the time of the study, a microwave system for controlled heating of small animal tumors was not commercially available. We therefore designed and constructed a temperature-controlled microwave system.

Development of hyperthermia equipment using microwaves for local tumor heating is a complicated task. It requires raising the temperature of a defined tissue volume to a predetermined level within a given time and maintaining that temperature with acceptable temperature gradients for a predetermined period. External microwave heating of a tumor in situ should be carried out uniformly without damaging the surrounding normal tissue. This demands precisely delivered, well-controlled, and accurately measured heating capabilities, which can adapt to the innate thermoregulatory subsystem of the complex biological system.

This paper describes a temperature-controlled microwave system operating at 2450 MHz, which is suitable for local heating of superficially growing small tumors in the rat. The principle of the system has been described elsewhere (Knöchel et al. 1982).

Recent Results in Cancer Research. Vol 101

Heating Equipment

The assembled microwave heating system is shown in Fig. 1. The system basically consists of a 2450-MHz, 250-W microwave generator (Philips MW127), which is modified for external power control, a temperature control unit, a small water-cooled direct contact applicator, a power meter, and a multichannel recorder. The microwave power is automatically pulsed. Temperature readings from the tumor at several locatations are carried out by microthermocouples at the end of the off periods of the generator. The influence of the microwave field on the temperature reading of the thermocouple will be described later. One of the thermocouples, the master probe, regulates the heating of the tumor via the control unit. For local hyperthermia studies, the tumor-bearing rats were under general anesthesia and were kept at a constant temperature level by thermostatically controlled water circulation (36.0° +/−0.1 °C).

The microwave power transferred to the tumor through the contact applicator is regulated by the control unit. The electrical design is shown in Fig. 2. Temperature measurement is performed in a bridge arrangement using the temperature of an electronic oven (Bailey Instruments Inc., United States, model OST-6 with NBS certificate) as reference. The actual temperature of the tumor is sampled at the shutoff period of the generator and is compared with the preset temperature value. The temperature difference is converted to a control signal which adjusts the amplitude of the next heating pulse. This is done by regulating the high voltage of the magnetron. A proportional-integral controller is additionally incorporated in the circuit in order to achieve a fast heating-up period of the tumor without errors in achieving the final temperature. The integral portion of the loop goes into operation as soon as 96% of the preset heating temperature is monitored. For a temperature of 43.0 °C, for example, control starts at 41.3 °C. The feedback of power-regulating signals in accordance with the temperature in the tumor leads to a fast initial increase in tumor temperature, followed by a well-defined temperature, which can be maintained within +/−0.1 °C during treatment. In the event of a temperature overshoot, the genera-

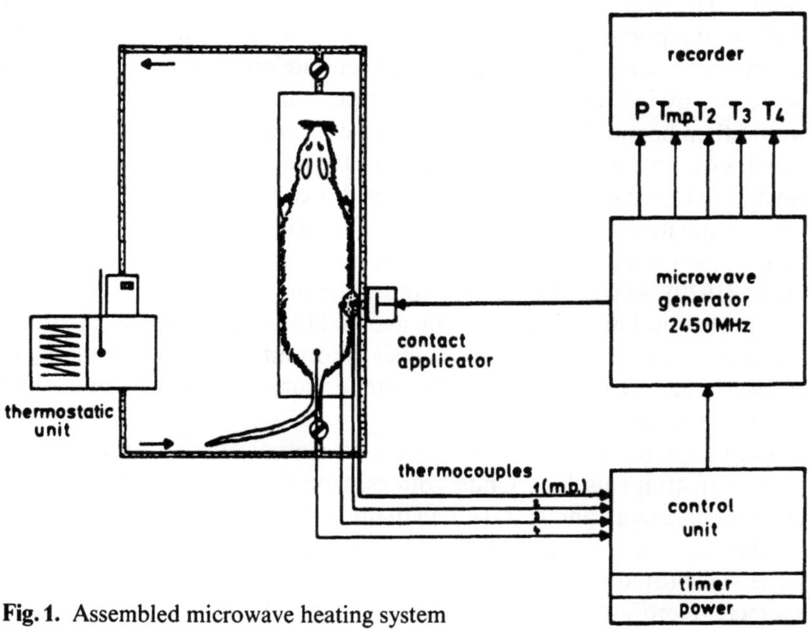

Fig. 1. Assembled microwave heating system

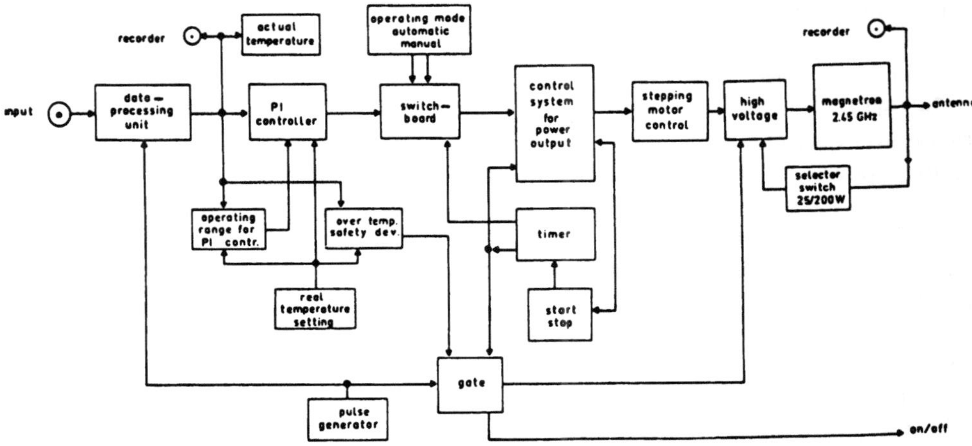

Fig. 2. Electrical design of the microwave heating system

tor is immediately switched off by the temperature safety device (0.2, 0.3, or 0.5 °C above the preset temperature). The control unit incorporates a timer circuit, which turns off the generator at the end of treatment.

The amplification of the control loop can be adjusted by means of the power on-power off ratio of the generator. Heating pulses of 2, 3, or 4 s can be selected; the time interval between two successive pulses is always 1 s. The various on-off ratios (2:1, 3:1, 4:1) were used to test the efficiency of various applicators with respect to local tumor heating.

Temperature Measurement

Tumor temperatures were measured using microthermocouples. Conventional needle probes incorporating thermistors or thermocouples cannot be used because they perturb the microwave field. A needle may concentrate on local fields and the metallic shaft can be heated by induced currents. The temperature of a tumor in the vicinity of the needle would then be much higher than if there were no probe. Thermocouples without metallic needles can be used in stationary microwave fields if they are oriented orthogonally to the electric field, which, in a tumor in situ, is difficult to achieve. In the case of a circularly polarized radiation field, the decoupling of the electromagnetic field and the thermocouple by orientation are even more complicated. It has been shown by Mendecki et al. (1978), Hand (1979), Magin (1979), and Bolmsjö et al. (1982) that interaction between temperature probes and microwaves can be avoided by using very small thermocouples or thermistors and by measuring temperatures at short intervals after switching off the microwave power. Under these conditions, the temperature read by a thermocouple corresponds to the tumor temperature.

The temperatures of the tumors were measured using implantable microthermocouples (Bailey Instruments Inc., United States, type IT-21). The thermocouple itself is made of copper constantan and is 200 μm in diameter; it has a sheath of Teflon (400 μm). Its length is 60 cm, its time constant 0.08 s. Each microthermocouple is previously calibrated in a large well-stirred water bath using a special clamp to hold it in front of a mercury thermometer (certified by the Deutsches Eichamt, Darmstadt, West Germany). Since the sta-

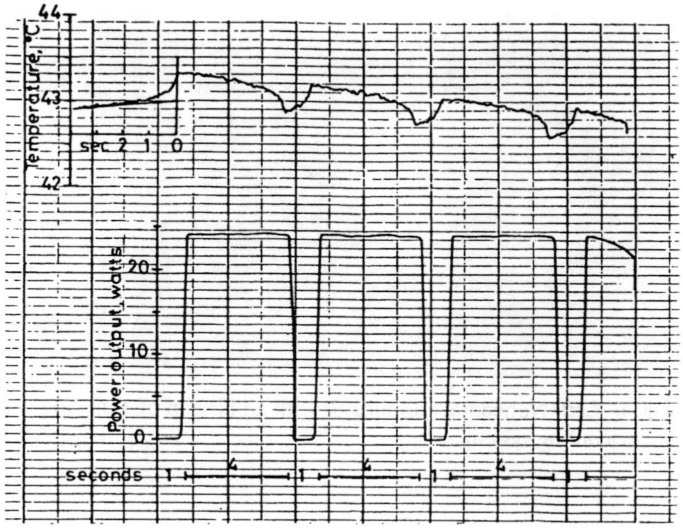

Fig. 3. Influence of microwave radiation on the temperature reading

bility of the reference temperature at 45 °C is better than 0.01 °C the accuracy of the temperature measurements is within +/−0.1 °C.

Microthermocouples were implanted in the tissue with removable 21-gauge needles and secured with surgical fibers. It was observed that the implantation of microthermocouples in the center of the tumor and their removal often led to bleeding from the tumor. The temperature reading of the probe then became erroneous. Therefore, in all experiments the master probe was implanted under the skin anterior to the tumor. The central location of the reference in the radiation field of the applicator also allowed relevant observations of the response of the skin.

The influence of microwave radiation on the temperature reading was studied by implanting a microthermocouple in the tumor. A spiral antenna for applying microwave power was used in the test. The result is shown in Fig. 3. In the presence of heating pulses of 4 s at a radiated power of 24 W, the temperature reading rises in accordance with the duration of the pulse. Once the power has been switched off, the temperature declines and rapidly approaches the temperature of the surrounding tissue. At 1 s after the power is switched off, the error of the recorded temperature value is +/−0.05 °C. In addition, the magnitude of field interaction is less when the radiated power is reduced.

Applicators

The applicator is a commercially available spiral antenna with circularly polarized radiation, which was designed for diathermy treatments (R. Bosch, Berlin, West Germany). This type of applicator has been described by Conway (1983). The applicator was used in two different ways: as a noncontact applicator with an air gap of 1 cm and as a direct-contact applicator with a water cooling system. The latter was temperature controlled by a thermocryostat (Haake, FRG, model F3-C digital) at 36.0+/−0.1 °C. Figure 4 shows the two applicators used.

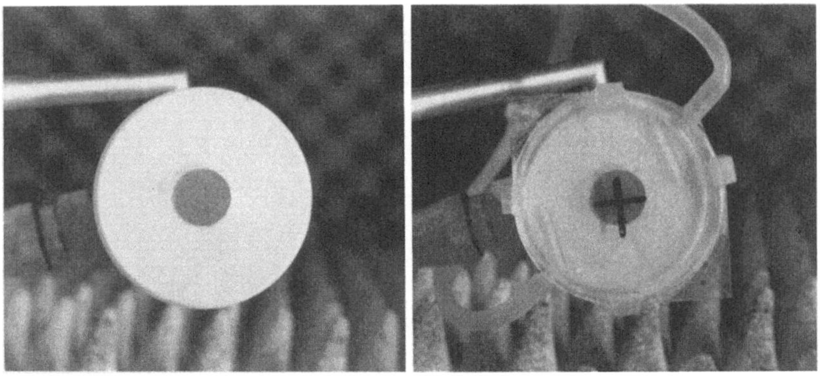

Fig. 4. *Left:* Noncontact applicator with an air gap of 1 cm. *Right:* Direct-contact applicator with a water-cooling system

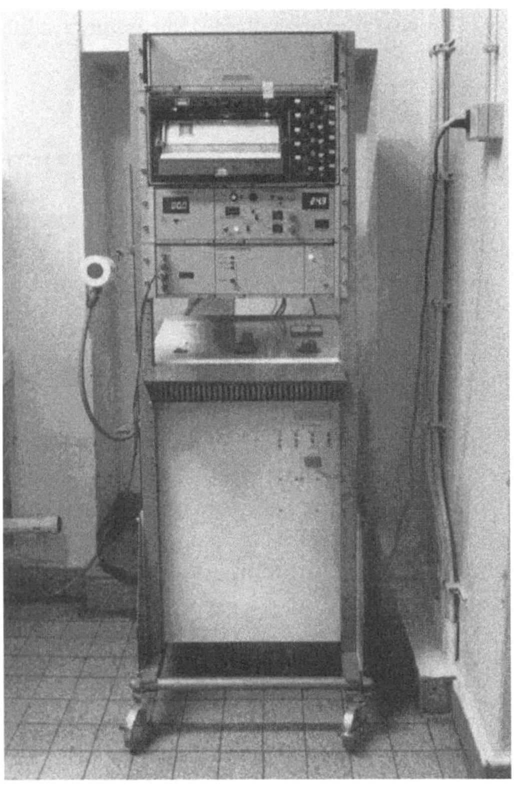

Fig. 5. Microwave hyperthermia system

Microwave Hyperthermia System

Figure 5 shows the microwave hyperthermia system. Technical data are listed in Table 1. The treatment temperature, the heating time, the on-off ratio of the power, and the safety threshold can be adjusted on the front panel of the control unit. During treatment, the radiated power or the reflection coefficient of the applicator and the temperature of the

Table 1. Technical details of the microwave hyperthermia system

Microwave generator
Frequency: 2450 MHz
Power output: 25, 50, and 250 W
Heating pulses: 2, 3, or 4 s
On-off ratios: 2:1, 3:1, or 4:1
External applicator
Contact spiral antenna with skin surface cooling, 6.5 cm in diameter
Temperature measurement
Microthermocouple
Copper constantan, 0.2 mm in diameter, with Teflon sheath, 0.4 mm in diameter
Time constant: 0.08 s
Bridge arrangement with electronic temperature reference, NBS certified
Accuracy: ±0.1 °C
Data storage
Multichannel recorder
Four temperatures
Radiated power

master probe are digitally displayed. The multichannel recorder on the top of the system registers the temperature profile of the master probe, the other three temperature profiles, and the radiated power during the course of treatment. In this way, each heated tumor is documented by the strip chart.

Local Hyperthermia of Rat Tumors

The microwave hyperthermia system was tested by heating solid rat tumors in a temperature range of 42.5-43.5 °C at various treatment times. The tumor was a rhabdomyosarcoma R1H superficially growing in the right flank of the animal. Details of the tumor assay have been described elsewhere (Jung et al. 1981). Tumors with volumes of 1.8 +/− 0.3 cm^3 and a diameter of 1.5 cm were selected for the temperature studies. Prior to treatment, the skin over the tumor was shaved. Heating by microwaves was performed in a shielded box. The rats were anesthetized with 6 mg/kg body weight xylazine hydrochloride (Rompun, Bayer) in combination with 50 mg/kg body weight ketamine hydrochloride (Ketanest, Parke-Davis). The weight of the animals was 240 +/− 10 g. Tumor and body temperature dropped by more than 1 °C as a result of anesthesia-induced hypothermia. A further decrease was stopped by positioning the animals in the temperature-controlled box.

Figure 6 shows an example of a typical registration for a rat tumor over a 60-min heating period. The time course of the master probe, of three other temperatures at different locations in the tumor, and of the radiated power are presented. At the beginning, the output of the generator was adjusted to approximately 28 W for about 2 min. This produced an increase in the tumor temperature of up to 41 °C at a rate of about 3 °C/min. At 41.3 °C the power control starts, thus achieving a smooth temperature profile of up to 43.0 °C. This temperature is automatically controlled every 5 s and is maintained within +/− 0.1 °C over the heating period. Once the desired tumor temperature is reached, the output power is continuously reduced and is lowered to 10 W by the end of the treatment. The temperature profiles of the thermocouples implanted in the center of the tumor or posterior to it show that heat is effectively and rapidly distributed throughout the whole

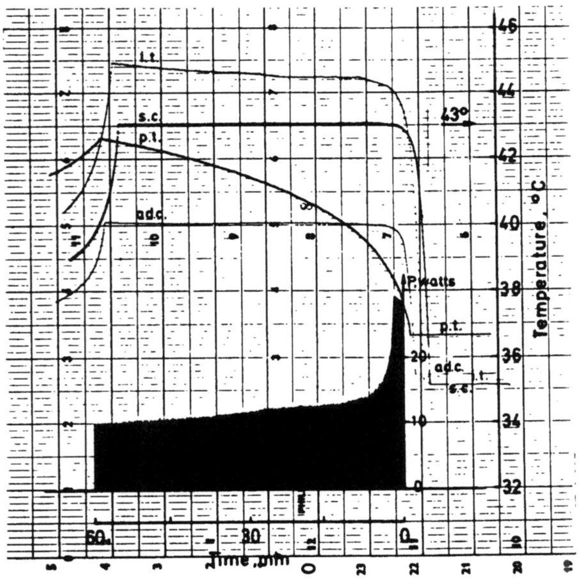

Fig. 6. Typical registration for a rat tumor over a 60-min heating period. Temperature monitoring on the skin *(ad c)*, under the skin *(sc)*, in the center *(it)*, and posterior to the tumor *(pt)*; *p*, radiated power

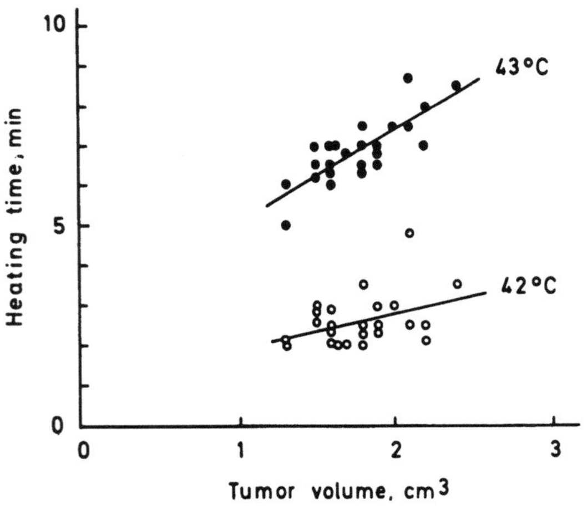

Fig. 7. Heating-up times for various tumor volumes

tumor, while the skin temperature is maintained at a level of about 40 °C. The temperature-time course of the master probe demonstrates that a system with amplitude-modulated heating pulses of constant length is advantageous compared with a system operating with variable pulse length modulation (Bolmsjö et al. 1982). Physical and biological changes that occur in the tumor tissue during treatment are rapidly compensated for with respect to the heating temperature.

Figure 7 shows heating-up times for various tumor volumes. It is obvious that larger tumors need longer to achieve the treatment temperature. Tumors of 1.8 + / − 0.3 cm^3, which were heated up to 43 °C within 6.6 + / − 1.2 min, had already exceeded 42 °C within 2.7 + / − 0.9 min after the beginning of treatment.

Temperature Distributions in Microwave-Heated Tumors

In a series of measurements, the temperature distribution in tumors heated by a noncontact and by a water-cooled contact applicator was investigated. For these experiments, three thermocouples were additionally implanted: one in the center of the tumor, one posterior to the tumor, and one in the rectum. It must be added that in the studies with the noncontact applicator the animals were placed on a Perspex holder without temperature stabilization. All hyperthermia runs were performed at 43.0 °C and 60 min. Nine tumors were heated with the noncontact applicator and 14 with the water-cooled contact applicator. Table 2 summarizes the mean temperature values at various times in the course of treatment.

The noncontact applicator takes about 9 min to heat the tumor to a temperature of 43.0 °C. The temperature in the center, i. e., at 0.8 cm tissue depth, is always higher than the adjusted skin temperature and finally exceeds that temperature by 0.8 °C. The temperature posterior to the tumor, i. e., at 1.5 cm depth, increases much more slowly. It takes more than 20 min to achieve the level of 42.0 °C, due to the poor penetration depth of 2450 MHz microwaves (Hahn et al. 1980; Lele 1980; Schwan 1980). Most of the radiated power is absorbed superficially, i. e., at less than 1 cm deep. The temperature distribution obtained with the water-cooled applicator (see Fig. 6, Table 2b) demonstrates that besides having shorter heating-up periods, the temperatures in the central and posterior portions of the tumor have analogous time courses but are generally somewhat higher than that with the noncontact applicator. Here, the maximum increase of temperature in the center of the tumor is 1.5 °C. The temperature at the posterior part of the tumor does not reach 43.0 °C; at the end of treatment 42.7 °C was measured. The rectal temperatures of the animals bearing

Table 2. Temperature values under the skin *(s. c.)*, in the center of the tumor *(i. t.)*, posterior to the tumor *(p. t.)*, and of the body of the rat *(rectal)* during microwave hyperthermia with two applicators at 43 °C for 60 min

Noncontact applicator

Locus	Start (°C)	Time (min)			
		9.2 ± 1.1	15.0	30.0	60.0
s. c.	30.3 ± 1.5	43.0 ± 0.1	43.0 ± 0.1	43.0 ± 0.1	43.0 ± 0.1
i. t.	31.5 ± 0.9	43.7 ± 0.8	43.6 ± 0.8	43.7 ± 0.7	43.8 ± 0.7
p. t.	31.6 ± 1.0	41.8 ± 1.0	41.9 ± 0.8	42.1 ± 0.7	42.2 ± 0.7
Rectal	33.5 ± 0.3	34.6 ± 0.6	35.1 ± 0.7	36.1 ± 0.9	37.0 ± 1.2

$n = 9$, $\bar{x} \pm SD$

Water-cooled contact applicator

Locus	Start (°C)	Time (min)			
		6.6 ± 1.2	15.0	30.0	60.0
s. c.	35.8 ± 0.4	43.0 ± 0.1	43.0 ± 0.1	43.0 ± 0.1	43.0 ± 0.1
i. t.	35.9 ± 0.5	43.6 ± 0.9	43.9 ± 0.9	44.2 ± 0.7	44.5 ± 0.7
p. t.	36.3 ± 0.4	40.6 ± 1.3	41.3 ± 1.2	42.1 ± 1.0	42.7 ± 0.7
Rectal	35.9 ± 0.4	36.1 ± 0.4	36.9 ± 0.6	38.4 ± 0.4	39.7 ± 0.3

$n = 14$, $\bar{x} \pm SD$

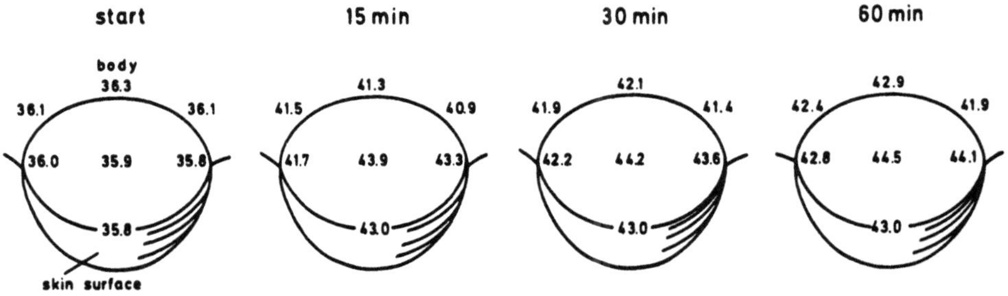

Fig. 8. Mapping of temperatures at all locations measured in a sectional plane through the middle of the tumor

tumors in the lower part of the body indicate an increase during treatment time. These temperatures accordingly are higher for the temperature-stabilized animals. At the end of treatment, rectal temperatures of about 40 °C were registered. This temperature was tolerated by the rats and there were no complications or deaths.

Further temperature studies were performed radial to the propagation direction of the radiation field at a depth of 0.8 cm and at a distance of 0.8 cm, and radial in the surrounding normal tissue at the posterior part of the tumor. The temperature profiles of 16 tumors that were comparable in volume and shape were evaluated. Figure 8 shows a mapping of temperatures at all locations measured in a sectional plane through the middle of the tumor. A continuous rise in temperature over the heating period is observed. The maximum temperature is obtained at 0.8 cm tissue depth. Thermal gradients exist at the radial distance to the center, which are different on the two sides of the tumor. For the part of the tumor close to the thigh of the rat, the gradient is steeper than for the opposite part near the abdominal wall. The temperature difference of 1.6 °C between these locations is reduced to 1.3 °C at the end of treatment. The temperatures posterior to the tumor also increase with treatment time but do not exceed temperature levels that damage the normal tissue (Storm et al. 1979).

Since the temperatures listed in Fig. 8 were obtained from different tumors, they are only indicative of the actual temperature gradients existing in any tumor of this size. It has to be noted that the temperature patterns are from tumors treated by microwaves for the first time. This pattern may change after multiple hyperthermic treatments due to physiological and morphological alterations in the tumor. The data indicate further that, even in an experimental tumor system, uniform heating is not being achieved. Besides the anatomical site of the tumor and the absorbed power distribution, the diffuse capillary blood flow and the main vessels are the most important factors that determine the temperature distribution in a tumor (Bicher et al. 1983; Song et al. 1980). The temperature distribution, however, is of great interest for the evaluation of tumor response after hyperthermic treatment (Dewhirst et al. 1984).

Conclusion

The technique of a 2450-MHz microwave system based on pulsed microwave radiation and temperature reading by microthermocouples has been described. The system permits an automated local heating of small animal tumors to predetermined temperature levels within predetermined treatment times. The adjustment of the temperature probe under the skin anterior to the tumor enables individual heating of each tumor to be carried out without producing significant whole body hyperthermia. The heating characteristics of the water-cooled contact applicator appear to make it of better therapeutic value than the noncontact applicator. Temperature profiles have been registered at different locations in the tumor and its surrounding normal tissue. Changes of intratumor temperatures with treatment time are observed. The system is currently being used to evaluate the therapeutic potential of localized hyperthermia as an adjuvant to radiotherapy in superficial rat tumors.

References

Bicher HI, Bruley DF (eds) (1982) Hyperthermia. Plenum, New York (Advances in experimental medicine, vol 157)

Bicher HI, Hetzel FW, Sandhu TS (1983) Physiology and morphology of tumour microcirculation in hyperthermia. In: Storm FK (ed) Hyperthermia in cancer therapy. GK Hall Medical Publishers, Boston, pp 207-222

Bolmsjö M, Hafström L, Hugander A, Jönsson PE, Persson B (1982) Experimental set-up for studies of microwave-induced hyperthermia in rats. Phys Med Biol 27: 397-406

Cheung AY (1982) Microwave and radiofrequency techniques for clinical hyperthermia. Br J Cancer [Suppl V]: 16-24

Christensen DA, Durney CH (1981) Hyperthermia production for cancer therapy: A review of fundamentals and methods. J Microwave Power 16: 89-105

Conway J (1983) Assessment of a small microwave (2450 MHz) diathermy applicator as suitable for hyperthermia. Phys Med Biol 28: 249-256

Dethlefsen LA (ed) (1982) Third International Symposium: Cancer Therapy by Hyperthermia, Drugs, and Radiation. Natl Cancer Inst Monogr 61

Dewey WC, Freeman ML (1980) Rationale for use of hyperthermia in cancer therapy. Ann NY Acad Sci 335: 372-378

Dewhirst MW, Sim DA, Sapareto S, Connor WG (1984) Importance of minimum tumour temperature in determining early and long-term responses of spontaneous canine and feline tumours to heat and radiation. Cancer Res 44: 43-50

Field SB, Bleehen NM (1979) Hyperthermia in the treatment of cancer. Cancer Treat Reviews 6: 63-94

Field SB, Streffer C (eds) (1982) Fourth Meeting of the European Co-operative Hyperthermia Group. Strahlentherapie 158: 378-392

Gauthérie M, Albert E (1982) Biomedical thermology, Liss, New York (Progress in clinical and biological research, vol 107)

Guy AW, Chou CK (1983) Physical aspects of localized heating by radiowaves and microwaves. In: Storm FK (ed) Hyperthermia in cancer therapy. GK Hall Medical Publishers, Boston, pp 270-304

Hahn GM (1982) Hyperthermia and cancer. Plenum, New York

Hahn GM, Kernahan P, Martinez A, Pounds D, Prionas S (1980) Some heat transfer problems associated with heating by ultrasound, microwaves or radiofrequency. Ann NY Acad Sci 335: 327-345

Hand JW (1979) A multi-channel system for microwave heating of tissues. Br J Radiol 52: 984-988

Hand JW, ter Haar G (1981) Heating techniques in hyperthermia. Br J Radiol 54: 443-466

Hill CR (ed) (1982) Proceedings of the Tenth LH Gray conference. Ultrasound, microwave and radiofrequency radiations: The basis for their potential in cancer therapy. Br J Cancer 45 [Suppl V]: 1-257

Hunt JW (1982) Applications of microwave, ultrasound, and radiofrequency heating. In: Dethlefsen LA (ed) Third International Symposium: Cancer Therapy by Hyperthermia, Drugs, and Radiation. Natl Cancer Inst Monogr 61: 447-456

Jain RK, Gullino PM (eds) (1980) Thermal characteristics of tumours: Applications in detection and treatment. Ann NY Acad Sci 335: 1-542

Jung H, Beck HP, Brammer I, Zywietz F (1981) Depopulation and repopulation of the R1H rhabdomyosarcoma of the rat after X-irradiation. Eur J Cancer 17: 375-386

Knöchel R, Meyer W, Zywietz F (1982) Dynamic in vivo performance of temperature controlled local microwave hyperthermia at 2.45 GHz. In: 1982 IEEE MTT-S International Microwave Symposium Digest, pp 444-447

Lele PP (1980) Induction of deep, local hyperthermia by ultrasound and electromagnetic fields. Radiat Environ Biophys 17: 205-217

Magin RL (1979) A microwave system for controlled production of local tumour hyperthermia in animals. IEEE Trans Microwave Theory Tech MTT 27: 78-83

Mendecki J, Friedenthal E, Botstein C, Sterzer F, Paglione R, Nowogrodzki M, Beck E (1978) Microwave induced hyperthermia in cancer treatment: Apparatus and preliminary results. Int J Radiat Oncol Biol Phys 4: 1095-1103

Milder JW (ed) (1979) Conference on hyperthermia in cancer treatment. Cancer Res 39: 2232-2340

Oleson JR, Dewhirst MW (1983) Hyperthermia: An overview of current progress and problems. Current problems in cancer. Year Book Medical Publishers, Chicago

Overgaard J (ed) (1984) Proceedings of the Fourth International Symposium on Hyperthermic Oncology. Taylor and Francis, London

Schwan HP (1980) Electromagnetic and ultrasonic induction of hyperthermia in tissue-like substances. Radiat Environ Biophys 17: 189-203

Song CW, Rhee JG, Levitt SH (1980) Blood flow in normal tissues and tumours during hyperthermia. JNCI 64: 119-124

Storm FK (ed) (1983) Hyperthermia in cancer therapy. GK Hall Medical Publishers, Boston

Storm FK, Harrison WH, Elliott RS, Morton DL (1979) Normal tissue and solid tumour effects of hyperthermia in animal models and clinical trials. Cancer Res 39: 2245-2251

Streffer C, van Beuningen D (eds) (1983) Fifth Meeting of the European Co-operative Hyperthermia Group. Strahlentherapie 159: 366-386

Zywietz F (1982) Effect of microwave heating on the radiation response of the rhabdomyosarcoma. Strahlentherapie 158: 255-257

An Automatic Hyperthermia System for Cancer Treatment

B. Audone, L. Bolla, and G. Marone

Aeritalia GEQ, Caselle Torinese, 10072 Torino, Italy

Introduction

The automatic system presented in this paper is based on a manual system, which was developed in collaboration with a team of physicians at the Molinette Hospital in Turin. The previous manual system had been used to perform trials and measurements on gel phantoms (aquasonic, polyacrylamide), for experiments in animals, and for clinical therapy in cancer patients. We then felt the need for a fully automatic system to ensure safe operating conditions, to avoid human errors, to standardize treatment protocol, and to record all relevant data of the treatment. A further goal was to avoid damage to the radiofrequency (RF) generators and apparatuses in the case of failures or human error (Audone et al. 1984).

System Description

The block diagram of the system is shown in Fig. 1. The computer is a 256-kbyte HP9816 with color CRT (cathode ray tube) monitor and color printer to display and record data during the treatment. The computer is interfaced with a multiprogrammer to control the apparatuses and to manage input/output operations.

The HF power is generated by three solid-state amplifiers operating in three different bands: (1) C-band (915 MHz), typical power 300 W; (2) B-band (434 MHz), typical power

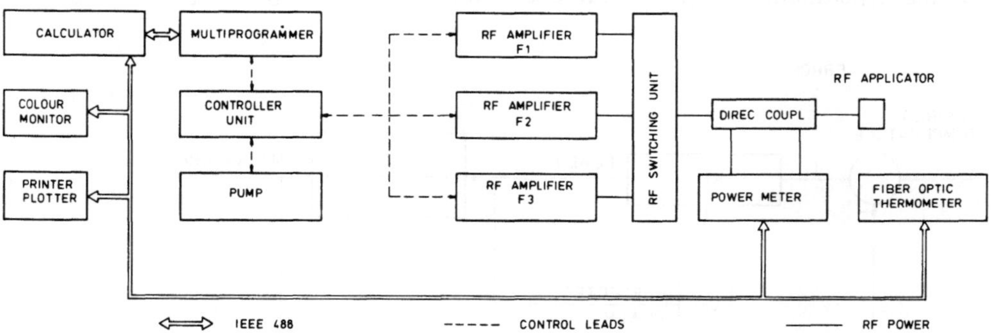

Fig. 1. Block diagram of an automatic system for hyperthermia cancer treatment

Recent Results in Cancer Research. Vol 101

300 W; and (3) A-band (2–30 MHz), typical power 500–700 W (frequency dependent); in the A-band the RF signal is generated by a 1-kHz stepped synthesizer, followed by a broad-band amplifier and an automatic tuner to match the generator to leads ranging from 10 to 300 ohms. The tuner is particularly useful in cases of loads with high reactive input impedance (e.g., capacitive electrodes), but may be bypassed using resonant antennas with minimal reactive components. The feedback signal is generated by a fiber optics four-channel Luxtron thermometer and by a power meter to measure incident and reflected power. The fiber optics thermometer has been chosen in place of other instruments (e.g., thermocouple, thermistor, high-resistivity thermistor) because it is the only one capable of operating correctly in the entire frequency range of interest without any susceptibility problem.

The system is composed of a cooling system with two independent circuits fed by a pump which controls the skin temperature ranging between 5 and 40 °C. This double cooling system makes it possible to differentiate the flow of the cooling liquid utilizing arrays of applicators or to cool large areas of the body using large antennae. Every parameter of the therapeutic treatment is displayed on the CRT color monitor, recorded on a floppy disk for data storage and presented on paper. A program has been added to the system to calculate in-depth thermal profiles in a multilayered biological structure. This program may thus be used as a starting point for comparative thermodosimetry.

Control Algorithm

The aim of hyperthermia therapy is to raise and to maintain at a fixed value the temperature of a certain volume of the human body affected by cancer. This control volume can be modeled as a first-order system, i.e., a system whose temperature response to a power step input is an exponential function (Fig. 2). The temperature is sampled at four points of interest chosen by the physician inside the control volume and one probe is selected as a main control probe. The real time measured temperature is compared with the desired temperature and the power delivered to the body is proportional to the difference between these values (error). Continuous power modulation has been chosen instead of on-off switching because of the minimal thermal tolerance required by hyperthermic treatment and to avoid dangerous thermal overshoots in healthy tissues. A theoretical temperature versus time curve (desired temperature) is compared with the temperature measured by the control probe; it is divided into two sections: during the transient stage (before reaching the hyperthermic range) the curve is a straight line passing through the origin, the

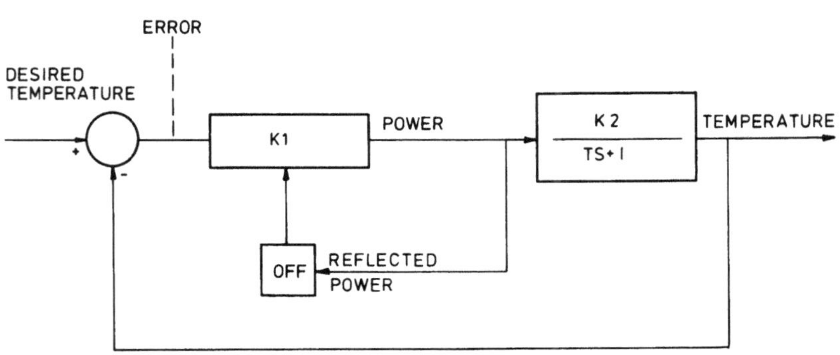

Fig. 2. Model of the control volume for hyperthermia therapy as a first-order system

slope of which is selected from three values by the operator. When the hyperthermic temperature is reached, the slope of the curve is zeroed and the measured temperature of the reference probe is allowed to oscillate $\pm 2\,^{\circ}C$ around the horizontal reference line. The choice of the transient slope is particularly delicate, because a warm-up that is too slow or thermal values that are too high could induce thermotolerance in cancer cells (Hahn 1984) which might abolish effectiveness of the therapy. Further safety controls are adopted for maximum and minimum temperature and for the VSWR (voltage standing wave ratio) value to warn the operator of possible antenna or probe-positioning error. Furthermore, to avoid delivering excessive power to small antennas, which could damage them, a code implemented in an electrical socket is assigned to each applicator. The applicator is recognized by the computer when the plug is inserted into the socket and if the antenna is not connected, no power can be delivered by the generator.

Thermal Model

A computer program has been developed and added to the system to solve the heat transfer partial derivatives differential equation or "bioheat" equation for a multilayered biological structure:

$$\rho c \frac{\delta T}{\delta t} = \nabla (k \nabla T) + Q_e + Q_m - Q_{bl} \tag{1}$$

where Q_e is the power density per volume unity generated by electromagnetic radiation, Q_m is the metabolic heat, and Q_{bl} is the heat dissipated by blood flow. The equation is solved in two steps:

1. Solution of the electromagnetic (EM) problem, i.e., the calculation of the dissipated EM power inside each layer, when a certain amount of incident power density on the first layer is given: the dissipated EM power is evaluated by means of the chained transmission matrix technique (Collin 1960; Nachmann and Turgeon 1984).
2. Solution of the thermal problem (it is assumed that the electrical properties of the tissues are not temperature dependent: $\delta\sigma/\delta T = 0$, $\delta E/\delta T = 0$) by means of a finite difference method (Strohben and Roemer 1984). The Q_m term for each tissue is temperature dependent, but its law of dependence is quite complex and many authors do not agree on its form (although some authors adopt an exponential model (van Sliedregt 1983). For these reasons we adopted an averaged value in the thermal range considered. As far as the Q_{bl} term is concerned, a satisfactory mathematical model to account for vasodilatation has not yet been found due to the nonlinearity occurring in this case. We thus chose a model such that the dissipated heat is proportional to the difference between the control volume temperature and the blood temperature, that is:

$$Q_{bl} = W_b C_b (T - T_b) \tag{2}$$

where W_b is the blood flow in volume per mass unity per time unity, C_b is the specific heat, and T_b is the blood temperature. The same kind of model has been adopted to evaluate the heat dissipation in the bolus by means of the cooling water flow. Equation (1) has been normalized and is solved in normalized spatial-temporal steps; the step amplitude is chosen to satisfy the stability condition.
The time required to calculate temperature profiles is then strongly dependent on the structure and ranges from about 5 calculated seconds per real second to 0.5 calculated second per real second (Figs. 3, 4).

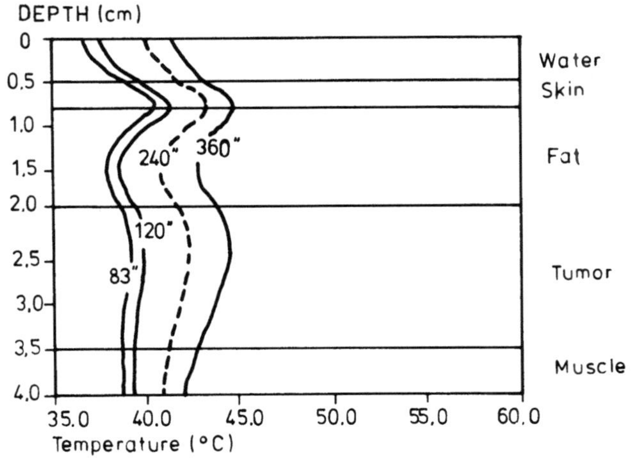

Fig. 3. Thermal profile without cooling bolus

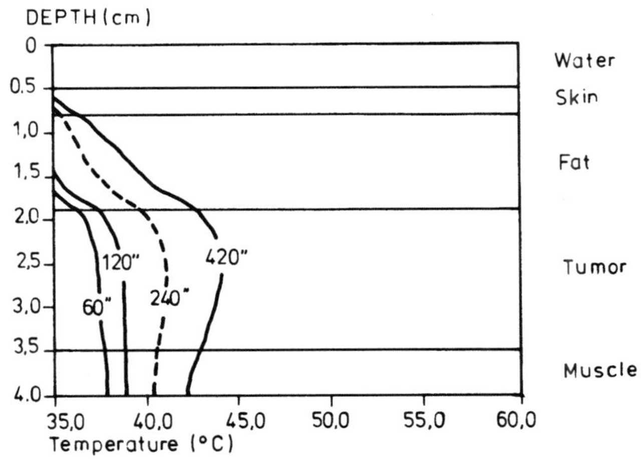

Fig. 4. Thermal profile with cooling bolus (Temp. 15 °C, water flux 0,5 l/min)

Applicators

Many kinds of applicators have been designed and tested for performance: ridged antenna (27 MHz), dielectric loaded rectangular waveguide antenna (433, 915 MHz), parallel rectangular waveguide antenna (915 MHz), and dipole antennas (interstitial and intracavitary). Inductive applicators are presently under study. The ridged antenna, which is about 30 × 70 cm, is filled with water to reduce its size and has been used to cure large tumors of the leg. Rectangular waveguides are filled with a ceramic material ($\varepsilon_r = 30$) and have been optimized to operate in contact with high dielectric constant materials.

We previously developed an applicator proposed by Guy (1978a, b); this applicator is made of two parallel rectangular waveguides filled with dielectric foamy material ($\varepsilon_r = 4$) and supplied by means of an inductive loop. This applicator has been adopted to meet the clinical needs of a square applicator: it has a heating area of approximately 13 × 13 cm and has reduced lateral radiation lobes to avoid excessive cutaneous heating. Thermal profiles in the lateral plane and in the transverse plane are reported in Figs. 5 and 6 for 14 W and 16 W of input power.

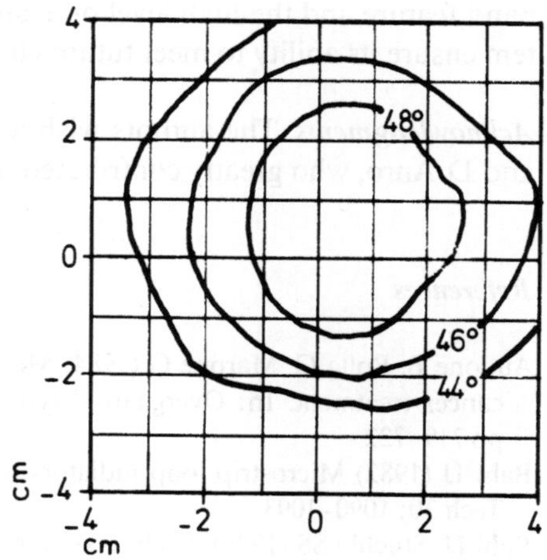

Fig. 5. Thermal profile in the lateral plane at 14 W of input power

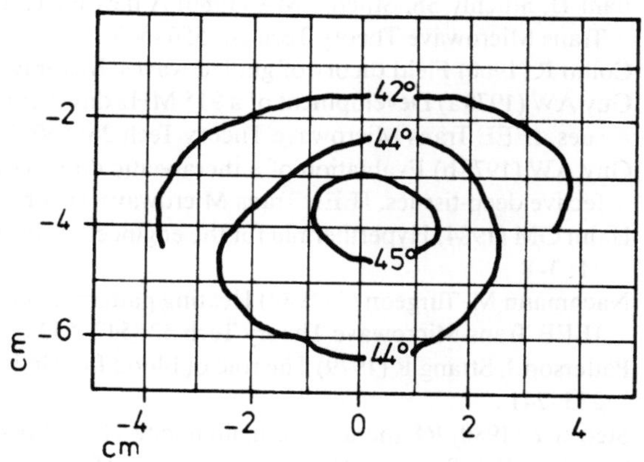

Fig. 6. Thermal profile in the transverse plane at 16 W of input power

Ring microstrip antennas utilize the TM_{210} mode, which is most suitable for its broadband feature and directivity (Bahl et al. 1980). The circular microstrip acts similar to a loaded (straight) microstrip line, whose characteristic impedance may be evaluated by means of a variational technique (Bahl and Stuchly 1980). The resonant frequency is evaluated using the semiempirical formula (Bahl 1982):

$$R \simeq \frac{6}{f\sqrt{|\varepsilon_r|}} \tag{3}$$

By adjusting the microstrip width, the input impedance of the antenna can be changed. The tuning is obtained by controlling its diameter and by means of a little stub installed on the opposite side of the connector. An array of three dipole antennae inserted inside after loading tubes has been designed for gynecological use and is now being tested.

Conclusions

The automatic hyperthermia system described above has been designed bearing in mind that this therapy is still under study and is in rapid and continuous evolution. It is therefore necessary to expect different kinds of applicators and arrays in the future. The broadband feature and the high level of available power with the modular structure of the system ensure its ability to meet future clinical needs.

Acknowledgments. The authors wish to express their gratitude to M. Francheo, L. Selmo, and D. Anrò, who greatly contributed to this work.

References

Audone B, Bolla G, Marone G (1984) Microwaves and RF computerized system for hyperthermic cancer treatment. In: Overgaard J (ed) Hyperthermic oncology. Taylor and Francis, London, pp 719-722

Bahl IJ (1982) Microstrip loop radiators for medical application. IEEE Trans Microwave Theory Tech 30: 1090-1093

Bahl IJ, Stuchly SS (1980) Analysis of a microstrip covered with a lossy dielectric. IEEE Trans Microwave Theory Tech 28: 1464-1468

Bahl IJ, Stuchly SS, Stuchly MA (1980) A new microstrip radiator for medical applications. IEEE Trans Microwave Theory Tech 26: 556-563

Collin R (1960) Field theory of guided waves. McGraw-Hill, New York, pp 76-87

Guy AW (1978a) Development of a 915 MHz direct contact applicator for therapeutic heating of tissues. IEEE Trans Microwave Theory Tech 26: 550-556

Guy AW (1978b) Evaluation of a therapeutic direct contact 915 MHz microwave applicator for effective deep-tissues. IEEE Trans Microwave Theory Tech 26: 556-563

Hahn GM (1984) Hyperthermia for the engineer: a short biological primer. IEEE Trans Biomed Eng 31: 3-8

Nachmann M, Turgeon G (1984) Heating pattern in a multilayered material exposed to microwaves. IEEE Trans Microwave Theory Tech 32: 547-552

Patterson J, Strang R (1979) The role of blood flow in hyperthermia. Int J Radiat Oncol Biol Phys 5: 235-241

Sterzer F (1980) RF therapy for malignancy. IEEE Spectrum 1980 Dec: 32-37

Strohben JW, Roemer RB (1984) A survey of computer simulations of hyperthermia treatments. IEEE Trans Biomed Eng 31: 136-149

Van Sliedregt M (1983) Computer calculation of a one-dimensional model, useful in the application of hyperthermia. Microwave J: 113-126

Hyperthermia System for Deep-Seated Tumors

G. Azam, G. Convert, J. Dufour, C. Jasmin, J. P. Mabire, L. Oweidat, and J. Sidi

CGR MeV, Filiale Thomson-CGR, Rue de la Minière, BP 34, 78530 Buc, France

In order to satisfy therapeutic needs in both oncology and infections pathology, CGR MeV (Thomson), has designed Jasmin 3-1000, a three electrode heating system which operates at 13.56 MHz.

A typical use of this equipment is heating of the pelvic region. In this case, the patient lies on a bed; an electrode is fitted under each buttock and a third electrode is placed above the pubis. Boluses filled with salinated water are inserted between the electrodes and the patient in close contact with the skin.

Principle of Operation

The system is interesting in that it allows the operator to control the distribution of energy deposition within the volume enclosed by the electrodes. The following brief description of the equipment and its mode of operation show how it is possible for this to be achieved.

A master oscillator drives three amplifiers with a nominal output power of 1 kW. Each of the amplifiers feeds one electrode through the inner conductor of a coaxial cable. The outer conductors are connected together at a common "neutral point." An attenuator and phase shifter circuits are inserted between the oscillator and the amplifiers.

Let $\mathbf{E}_1$, $\mathbf{E}_2$, $\mathbf{E}_3$ be a three-vector system representing the relative amplitudes and phases at the electrodes ($|\mathbf{E}_n|^2$ measures the power applied to the electrode n). Circuits allow defi-

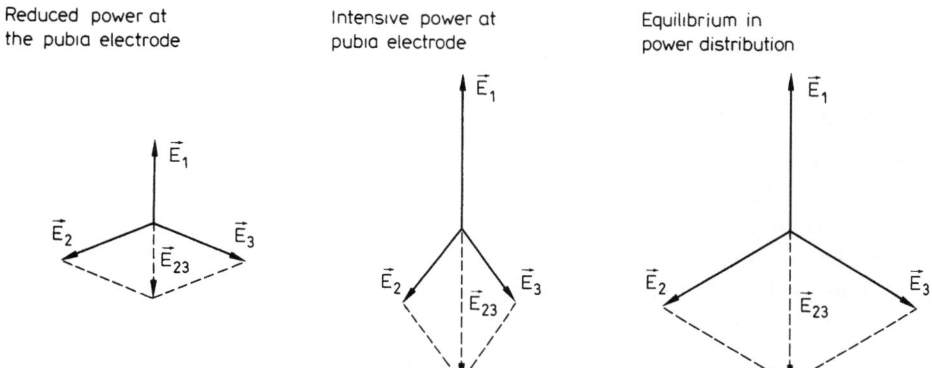

Fig. 1. Different vectorial configurations: theoretical presentation

Recent Results in Cancer Research. Vol 101

nition of $\mathbf{E}_3$ as equal to the vectorial sum ($\mathbf{E}_2+\mathbf{E}_3$). This means that no power can flow through the neutral point, so that each amplifier can be matched to its load as if it were alone. Furthermore, by adjusting the phase ρ_3 between $\mathbf{E}_2$ and $\mathbf{E}_3$ (see Fig. 1), we can control the power applied to electrode 1 and, as a consequence, the distribution of energy deposition throughout the heated volume.

On the other hand, the peripheral temperature of the heated region can be controlled by adjusting the temperature and the flow of the water within the boluses.

Phantom Tests

Jasmin 3-1000 was tried out on phantoms before any clinical testing was carried out. The total volume heated was about 18 liters.

The objective of these tests was to evaluate the distribution of energy deposition. This was achieved by measuring the temperature increase in an array of alcohol thermometers inserted inside the phantom. The distribution is proportional to the temperature increase provided the heating time is not too long.

The tests have shown that a fairly homogeneous distribution can be achieved with the equipment.

Clinical Applications

Phase A clinical trials were first carried out to evaluate the tolerance and the toxicity of hyperthermia treatments with Jasmin 3-1000. This equipment was used both for the treatment of malignant tumors and for the treatment of venereal diseases.

Patient Comfort

The aim is to operate in conditions which avoid burns with near 100% certainty. On the other hand, the electromagnetic radiation must be kept at a very low level to avoid discomfort to the patient.

Protocol Selected After Clinical Trials

The protocol established after the preliminary trials is as follows:

1. Each session lasts 60–90 min, including heating-up time
2. Heating-up takes 20–30 min, according to patients and their body type
3. Water cooling is supplied to prevent skin temperatures from exceeding 42–43 °C
4. The therapeutic temperature selected is 41–41.5 °C in the case of infectious diseases, and above 42 °C in the case of malignant tumors. It has been observed that these temperatures can be maintained for about 30 min with no discomfort to the patient.

In our trials, the mean power applied was in the range of 500–600 W, according to the volume to be heated.

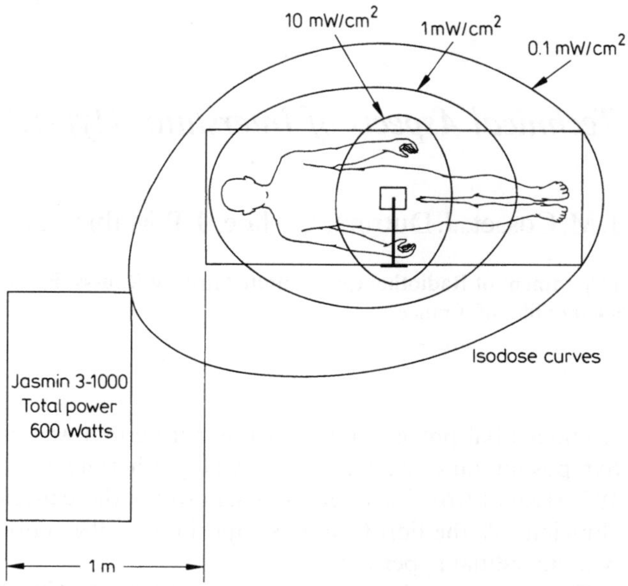

Fig. 2. Electromagnetic radiation measurement (mW/cm^2). Radiation is 10 mW/cm^2 50 cm above the pubis and 30 cm below the bed. Outside the isodose 0.1 mW/cm^2 radiation is negligible

Thermometry

Vaginal and rectal temperatures were measured with alcohol thermometers. Intratumoral measurements were performed during the treatment sessions by means of a noninterfering electronic thermometer designed at CGR MeV (patent pending).

Electromagnetic Radiation

Due to a careful design for matching of the amplifiers to their load, the electromagnetic radiation is kept to a very low level. The electromagnetic isodoses noted in Fig. 2 show that the main part of the body lies outside the area defined by the admitted tolerance value. The physicians and their assistants are exposed to doses 100 lower than this tolerance value. The radiation involves no discomfort to patients or staff.

Conclusion

As pointed out above, the tests we carried out focused particularly on the questions of tolerance and toxicity during hyperthermia treatments in the course of which large volumes were heated.

The temperatures aimed at were 41 °C for 45 min for the treatment of venereal diseases and 42 °C for 20 min for the treatment of malignant tumors. These temperatures have been achieved and maintained with no difficulty in all 35 sessions so far completed.

At the same time, no alarming changes have been recorded in oral temperature, skin temperature, pulse rate, or blood pressure during or after the treatment.

Technical Aspects of Interstitial Hyperthermia

J. M. Cosset, J. Dutreix, C. Haie, J. P. Mabire, and E. Damia

Department of Radiotherapy, Institute Gustave Roussy, Rue Camille Desmoulins, 94800 Villejuif, France

An interstitial procedure for local hyperthermia was proposed at the First International Symposium on Cancer Therapy by Hyperthermia, which was held in Washington DC in 1975 (Doss 1976). For several years, however, these invasive techniques seemed to frighten clinicians. At the Fort Collins Symposium in 1980, only a limited number of papers dealt with interstitial hyperthermia.

Due to encouraging preliminary results obtained in a few centers, and perhaps to disappointments in some "external" techniques, interest in interstitial procedures is now rapidly growing. At the international Aarhus meeting held in Denmark in July 1984, 20 posters were presented concerning invasive hyperthermia.

In this technical paper, we shall essentially study the two main techniques which are presently in use in Europe, in Japan, and in the United States.

Radiofrequency Technique

The radiofrequency (RF) technique utilizes resistive heating by means of RF electric currents driven between pairs of implanted electrodes. The frequency is usually in the range of 0.5-1 MHz (Cosset et al. 1984a, b; Emami et al. 1984; Joseph et al. 1981; Le Bourgeois et al. 1978; Lilly et al. 1983; Manning et al. 1982; Visser et al. 1984; Vora et al. 1982; Yabumoto and Suyama 1984). Different types of amplifiers have been proposed.

A minimum available power of 25 W for each pair of electrodes seems necessary. In most modern generators, the power can be adjusted for each implanted probe, with a safety device preventing the temperature from reaching a preset value.

The optimal material to be implanted is still under discussion. When RF currents are used, perfect contact between the metallic probe and tissues is mandatory. Thus the most "classical" material for implantation is a set of metallic needles directly connected to the generator. Although these needles heat safely and correctly (Emami et al. 1984; Joseph et al. 1981; Lilly et al. 1983; Manning et al. 1982; Visser et al. 1984; Vora et al. 1982; Yabumoto and Suyama 1984), some drawbacks have recently been pointed out. First, this rigid material is not very well tolerated by the patient, not only during the hyperthermia session, but also during the usual posthyperthermia brachytherapy period (several days). Secondly, the heat is not only delivered to the tumor but also to some volume of normal surrounding tissues and to the skin surface at the entry and exit sites.

Recent Results in Cancer Research. Vol 101

To overcome the unnecessary heating of normal structures, and knowing that insulation is easily achieved at a frequency of 0.5–1 MHz, two centers (Stanford, United States, and Paris, France, Cosset et al. 1984a, b) developed special "metallic plastic" tubes. The length of a central metallic portion is individualized for each tumor; the two plastic parts on each side make possible perfect insulation of the normal tissues. The RF power is transmitted to the metallic portion by means of a specially designed probe, inserted into the plastic end until it contacts the metallic part. With this technique, the tumor can be heated while the skin and the normal surrounding tissues are almost completely spared.

These special tubes can be loaded with iridium 192 wires after or before the hyperthermia session, to be used for brachytherapy.

Some guidelines should be kept in mind regarding the geometry of the implantation:

1. The distance between the two electrodes of a pair should not exceed 15 mm to avoid a "cold spot" at mid-distance between the probes. The optimum spacing is 10–15 mm. The distance between two pairs of electrodes for correct distribution of both temperature and irradiation dose is likely to be the same as that between the electrodes. Moreover, this technique makes possible a "rearrangement" of the connections, which is sometimes necessary to improve the temperature distribution.
2. The parallelism of the electrodes must be perfect, in order to avoid "cold" or "hot" spots.
3. The length of the two electrodes of a pair should be approximately the same. If not, in spite of the individualized regulation of the power, this can lead to an "overheating" of the shorter probe.
4. Interstitial hyperthermia techniques facilitate the thermometry procedure, since thermal probes can be inserted in the various heating lines. Complete thermal mapping is thus possible. In order to improve this assessment of the temperature distribution, additional plastic catheters are sometimes inserted in the tumors, which is essential to evaluate the minimum temperature reached in the heated volume. With RF currents, a complete thermal recording can be obtained throughout the hyperthermia session, since interference seldom disturbs thermocouples or thermistors.

Microwave Technique

The microwave technique utilizes radiative heating by means of coaxial microwave antennae. The frequency varies from 300 to 915 MHz (Arcangeli et al. 1982; Bicher et al. 1984a, b; Coughlin et al. 1984; Emami et al. 1984; Gidman et al. 1984a, b; Lev et al. 1984; Luk et al. 1984; Nussbaum et al. 1984; Roos and Hamnerieus 1984; Syed et al. 1984; Trembly et al. 1984; Wong et al. 1984). Different types of generators are available, all of which allow individualized regulation of the power in each implanted antenna.

The choice of material for implantation is less problematic than for RF techniques. At a frequency of 300–1000 MHz, the plastic tubes are no longer capable of insulating, and therefore the classical plastic carriers used for brachytherapy applications can be utilized. The coaxial microwave antennae are inserted in each plastic tube. The heating "length" is the same as that of the antenna. The clinician, therefore, must have a wide range of antennae available, with different lengths to adapt the technique to the tumor. This poses a major problem for large tumors, which need 10- to 15-cm antennae (not yet available).

The geometry is not limited by the fact that one must work with pairs of electrodes, as in the RF current technique. Each antenna emits separately. Theoretically, the spacing of the electrodes can reach 20-25 mm with an acceptable temperature distribution. But in the clinic, it is not advisable to use spacing of more than 15 mm for two reasons:

1. An unpredictable high blood flow rate or change in tissue conductivity can lead to large temperature inhomogeneities in some instances
2. This is the normal spacing used for the brachytherapy application (which is combined with interstitial hyperthermia in almost all cases)

The parallelism must be as perfect as for the RF technique, for the same reasons as those detailed above.

Concerning thermometry, we must remember that interferences can occur with "classical" thermometers such as thermocouples or ordinary thermistors. When utilizing these thermal probes, the temperature reading has to be made after switching off the power. But the best solution is to use noninterferent temperature probes, such as fiber optic or Bowman's probes.

Future Directions

In spite of the recent and rapid developments of interstitial techniques for hyperthermia, not all of the technical problems have been solved. In most cases, either RF or microwave interstitial procedures can achieve, in the present state of the art, a homogeneous heating at a therapeutic level (43°-44 °C) in a well-defined volume. But in some cases, the temperature distribution is disappointing, even with a perfect implantation geometry.

Temperature inhomogeneities up to 2°-3 °C have been observed in the heated tumor (Cosset et al. 1984a, b). This is probably due to unpredictable large inhomogeneities of the tissue conductivities and/or to variations of the blood flow rate (Strohben 1983; Chan et al. 1984). We observed, for example, that it was impossible to reach more than 41 °C very close to a small artery, even with a perfect application. This emphasizes the need for precise thermometry that is able to provide complete temperature mapping of the heated tumor. These results allow the power to be regulated in each line in order to obtain an acceptable temperature distribution compromise.

While most of the groups involved in interstitial hyperthermia are working to improve RF or microwave procedures (with which they have treated about 200 patients all over the world), some others are working in a totally different way, looking for other solutions for invasive hyperthermia. At the Universities of Arizona and of Alabama, a totally new procedure is under study. Ferromagnetic seeds are implanted in the tumors and are then heated by a high-frequency magnetic field. Recently, newly designed self-regulating thermoseeds have prevented the temperature from reaching a value higher than the seed's Curie point. This new technique has already been tested in spontaneous tumors in pet animals, with encouraging preliminary results (Atkinson and Brezovich 1984; Deshmukh et al. 1984; Forsyth et al. 1984; Manning and Gerner 1983). A drawback of this method is the fact that it cannot be easily combined with brachytherapy (but it can be combined with external irradiation). However, this technique makes it possible to treat some sites we cannot easily implant with the "classical" material for radiofrequency or microwave heating, especially deep-seated tumors. This new technique clearly deserves further development and clinical evaluation.

Conclusion

Interstitial RF or microwave hyperthermia techniques presently enable clinicians to reach a significant temperature (43° - 44 °C, minimum) homogeneously in mostly well-defined tumor volumes. Technical developments are still necessary for the treatment of tumors and also to avoid temperature inhomogeneities that occur in some cases.

New procedures for interstitial hyperthermia such as the self-regulating inductively heated thermoseeds deserve further evaluation.

References

Arcangeli G, Barni E, Cividalli A, Lovisolo G, Nervi C, Mauro F (1982) Hyperthermia by implantable applicators. In: Gautherie M (ed) Biomedical thermology. Liss, New York, pp 641-647

Atkinson WJ, Brezovich IA (1984) Interstitial heating of tumors by thermally self regulating nickel-copper seeds. Abstracts of the 4th International Symposium on Hyperthermic Oncology, Aarhus, Denmark, July 2-6, D 10

Bicher HI, Wolfstein RS, Fingerhut AG, Frey HS, Lewinsky BS (1984a) An effective fractionation regime for interstitial thermoradiotherapy - preliminary clinical results. In: Overgaard J (ed) Hyperthermic oncology, vol 1. Taylor and Francis, London, pp 575-578

Bicher HI, Moore DW, Wolfstein RS (1984b) A method for interstitial thermoradiotherapy. In: Overgaard J (ed) Hyperthermic oncology, vol 1. Taylor and Francis, London, pp 595-598

Chan KW, Miller W, Roemer RB, Williamson J, Cetas TC (1984) Thermal dosimetry of RF interstitial hyperthermia. Abstracts of the 4th International Symposium on Hyperthermic Oncology, Aarhus, Denmark, July 2-6, D2

Cosset JM, Brule JM, Salama AM, Damia E, Dutreix J (1982) Low-frequency (0.5 MHz) contact and interstitial techniques for clinical hyperthermia. In: Gauthérie M (ed) Biomedical thermology. Liss, New York, pp 649-657

Cosset JM, Dutreix J, Dufour J, Janoray P, Damia E, Haie C, Clarke D (1984a) Combined interstitial hyperthermia and brachytherapy: Institute Gustave-Roussy technique and preliminary results. Int J Radiat Oncol Biol Phys 10: 307-312

Cosset JM, Dutreix J, Gerbaulet A, Damia E (1984b) Combined interstitial hyperthermia and brachytherapy: the Institute Gustave-Roussy experience. In: Overgaard J (ed) Hyperthermic oncology, vol 1. Taylor and Francis, London, pp 587-590

Coughlin CT, Roberts DW, Wong TZ, Strohbein JW, Douple EB, Colacchio TA (1984) Clinical experience with deep seated intra-abdominal and brain tumors using an interstitial microwave antenna array for hyperthermia. Abstracts of the 4th International Symposium on Hyperthermic Oncology, Aarhus, Denmark, July 2-6, D 15

Deshmukh R, Damento M, Demer L, Forsyth K, Deyoung J, Dewhirst M, Cetas TC (1984) Ferromagnetic alloys with Curie temperatures near 50 °C for use in hyperthermic therapy. In: Overgaard J (ed) Hyperthermic oncology, vol 1. Taylor and Francis, London, pp 571-574

Doss JD (1976) Use of RF fields to produce hyperthermia in animal tumors. In: Robinson JE (ed) Proceedings of the international symposium on cancer therapy by hyperthermia and radiation. American College of Radiology, Washington, p 226

Emami B, Marks J, Perez C, Nussbaum G, Leybovich L (1984) Treatment of human tumors with interstitial irradiation and hyperthermia. In: Overgaard J (ed) Hyperthermic oncology, vol 1. Taylor and Francis, London, pp 583-586

Forsyth K, Deshmukh R, Deyoung DW, Dewhirst M, Cetas TC (1984) Recent clinical experience in pet animals with hyperthermic therapy in the head and neck region induced with inductively-heated ferromagnetic implants. In: Overgaard J (ed) Hyperthermic oncology, vol 1. Taylor and Francis, London, pp 599-602

Gidman V, Roos D, Lindskoug BA (1984a) Intercomparison of microwave antennas for hyperthermia. Abstracts of the 4th International Symposium on Hyperthermic Oncology, Aarhus, Denmark, July 2-6, D4

Gidman V, Notter G, Lindskoug BA (1984b) Interstitial hyperthermia using mobile antennas as an adjuvant to interstitial afterloading of a mobile Ir-192 source for high dose rate radiotherapy. Abstracts of the 4th International Symposium on Hyperthermic Oncology, Aarhus, Denmark, July 2-6, D20

Joseph CD, Astrahan M, Lipsett J, Archambeau J, Forell B, George FW (1981) Interstitial hyperthermia and interstitial iridium-192 implantation: a technique and preliminary results. Int J Radiat Oncol Biol Phys 7: 827-833

Le Bourgeois JP, Convert G, Dufour J (1978) An interstitial device for microwave hyperthermia of human tumors. In: Streffer C (ed) Cancer therapy by hyperthermia and radiation. Urban and Schwarzenberg, Munich, pp 122-124

Lev A, Lieb Z, Servadio C, Shtrikman S, Treves D (1984) Heat profiles of 915 MHz skirt-type antenna. Abstracts of the 4th International Symposium on Hyperthermic Oncology, Aarhus, Denmark, July 2-6, D8

Lilly MB, Brezovich IA, Atkinson W, Chakraborty D, Durant JR, Ingram J, McElvein R (1983) Hyperthermia with implanted electrodes. In vitro and in vivo correlations. Int J Radiat Oncol Biol Phys 9: 373-382

Luk KH, Jiang HB, Chou CK (1984) SAR patterns of a helical microwave intracavitary applicator. In: Overgaard J (ed) Hyperthermic oncology, vol 1. Taylor and Francis, London, pp 591-594

Manning MR, Gerner EW (1983) Interstitial thermoradiotherapy. In: Storm FK (ed) Hyperthermia in cancer therapy. Hall, Boston

Manning MR, Cetas TC, Miller RC, Oleson JR, Connor WG, Gerner EW (1982) Clinical hyperthermia: results of a phase I trial employing hyperthermia alone or in combination with external beam. Cancer 49: 205-216

Nussbaum GH, Leibovich LB, Emami B, Perez CA, Johnston R, Straube WL (1984) Techniques for improved administration of interstitial hyperthermia with microwaves. Abstracts of the 4th International Symposium on Hyperthermic Oncology, Aarhus, Denmark, July 2-6, D3

Roos D, Hamnerieus Y (1984) Development of a microwave applicator for intracavitary hyperthermia treatment. Abstracts of the 4th International Symposium on Hyperthermic Oncology, Aarhus, Denmark, July 2-6, D6

Strohben JW (1983) Temperature distributions from interstitial RF electrode hyperthermia systems: theoretical predictions. Int J Radiat Oncol Biol Phys 9: 1655-1667

Syed AMN, Puthawala AA, Sheikh KMA (1984) Microwave interstitial hyperthermia in the management of extensive primary and recurrent tumors. Abstracts of the 4th International Symposium on Hyperthermic Oncology, Aarhus, Denmark, July 2-6, D16

Trembly BS, Richter HJ, Mechling JA (1984) The effect of antenna surface cooling on the temperature distribution of an interstitial microwave antenna array. Abstracts of the 4th International Symposium on Hyperthermic Oncology, Aarhus, Denmark, July 2-6, D7

Visser AG, Martina HJ, van Rhoon GC (1984) RF interstitial hyperthermia: phantom measurements and computer simulations for different needle configurations. Abstracts of the 4th International Symposium on Hyperthermic Oncology, Aarhus, Denmark, July 2-6, D1

Vora N, Forell B, Joseph C, Lipsett J, Archambeau JO (1982) Interstitial implant with interstitial hyperthermia. Cancer 50: 2518-2523

Yabumoto E, Suyama S (1984) Interstitial radiofrequency hyperthermia in combination with external beam radiotherapy. In: Overgaard J (ed) Hyperthermic oncology, vol 1. Taylor and Francis, Londons pp 579-582

Wong TZ, Strohbehn JW, Smith KF, Trembly BS, Douple EB, Coughlin CT (1984) An interstitial microwave antenna array system (IMAAH) for local hyperthermia. Abstracts of the 4th International Symposium on Hyperthermic Oncology, Aarhus, Denmark, July 2-6, D9

Ultrasound-Induced Hyperthermia

Introduction

H. D. Kogelnik

Institut für Radiotherapie, Landeskrankenanstalten Salzburg, Müllner Hauptstrasse 48,
5020 Salzburg, Austria

Ultrasound offers special advantages in the heating of both superficial and deep-seated soft tissues. This is because of its flexibility and its ability to focus the beam onto the target region.

Ultrasound-induced hyperthermia has been used for many decades in the treatment of cancer. One of the earliest reports appeared in the German literature 40 years ago, describing its effect on a human sarcoma (Dyroff 1944). However, because of excessive heating, particularly near bone interfaces, with resulting elevated temperatures in bone, this heating method had not often been used until recently.

Over the past few years, a great deal of research has been done on the specific physical properties of ultrasound in soft tissues. As a result, and because of the development of new focusing devices, ultrasound is now increasingly used at the clinical level. There are about 15–20 major centers worldwide involved in ultrasound-induced hyperthermia for cancer treatment, and several clinical pilot studies are in progress.

Why ultrasound holds so much promise for therapeutic heating is because it provides easy generation of heat and possesses good localization properties. Ultrasound frequencies from about 0.3 to 3.0 MHz are used for tissue heating. In soft tissue, a frequency of 1 MHz leads to a wavelength of only 2.5 mm.

Short wavelength and good penetration are unique features of ultrasound. Because of the short wavelength of therapeutically useful ultrasound, well-defined beams can be produced by transducers with diameters of only a few centimeters. A coupling medium, usually water contained behind a very flexible thin latex membrane, is needed between the transducer and the skin. By adjusting the water temperature, skin temperature can be controlled. Ultrasonic gel is used to ensure optimal coupling of the water jacket to the skin. In this way, a continuous medium for the efficient propagation of the sound waves is established.

Because of interference effects within the near field of a propagating wave, large variations in the local field intensity are caused. This near-field zone extends to the treated tissue, where blood flow and thermal conduction smooth out most of these intensity variations.

Only superficial tumors can be heated, with plane transducers in the form of circular disks. For selective heating at depth, besides using the more penetrating lower frequencies, geometric gain has to be added by a combination of focusing, scanning, or the simultaneous use of multiple transducers.

Recent Results in Cancer Research. Vol 101

Several centers are developing instrumentation to combine focusing and scanning for preferential deep heating. The automated scanning equipment used by Lele et al. (1983) allows for varying the average energy deposition three-dimensionally, which results in very favorable and uniform temperature distributions at these depths. A clinical limitation of scanning when heating larger tissue volumes might be the cooling that occurs in this region during the time that no power is applied. Large tissue volumes may need a certain time before the scanning pattern repeats, and during this time blood flow and thermal conduction can cause significant cooling of the tissue of interest.

Focusing and scanning can also be accomplished electronically by manipulation of relative phases. However, as yet no systems have been developed for clinical investigations.

The use of several transducers simultaneously is a direct way of incorporating geometric gain for selective heating of deep-seated tumors. In the original version of a system developed at Stanford, six transducers operating at about 0.35 MHz were mounted on the inside of a spherical shell (Hahn et al. 1981). The geometric focus can thus be positioned to a depth of up to 15 cm below the skin surface.

Major disadvantages of ultrasound include its high absorption in bone and its reflection at tissue interfaces. The absorption of ultrasound in bone is much greater than in soft tissue, which results in the excessive heating of superficial layers of bone. Of the soft tissues, attenuation values in fat are lower than in muscle. Therefore, a higher temperature is expected in muscle, but a much higher one in bone.

With ultrasound, there is a nearly 100% reflection at the soft tissue/air interface and about a 40% reflection at a soft tissue/bone interface. Clinically, therefore, there are restrictions assigned to ultrasound-induced hyperthermia for tumors in the lungs or when bone is in the close vicinity of the tumor. In spite of these restrictions, ultrasound is an important alternative approach to tissue heating, mainly because of the excellent temperature distribution which is achievable at depth.

References

Dyroff R (1944) Ultraschallwirkung beim menschlichen Sarkom. Strahlentherapie 75: 126

Hahn GM, Marmor JB, Pounds D (1981) Induction of hyperthermia by ultrasound. Bull Cancer (Paris) 68: 249

Lele PP (1983) Physical aspects and clinical studies with ultrasonic hyperthermia. In: Storm FK (ed) Hyperthermia in cancer therapy. Hall, Boston, pp 333-367

Theoretical and Technical Aspects of the Design of Ultrasonic Hyperthermia Equipment

E. G. Lierke

Battelle-Institut, Abteilung für Physikalische Technik und Bauelemente, Am Römerhof 35, 6000 Frankfurt/Main, FRG

Introduction

Parallel to research and development work in other countries (Lele 1983; Hynynen et al. 1982), in 1980 the German Ministry for Research and Technology (BMFT) initiated a research and development on study local hyperthermia with ultrasonics of superficial and deep-located tumors. The two main objectives of the first phase of the study were:

1. Identification and evaluation of the primary physiological and technical parameters essential for optimizing ultrasonic equipment and treatment procedures, including therapeutic risks
2. Construction and assessment of an optimized ultrasonic facility (engineering model) for later clinical application

The investigations had to be based on the state of the art in ultrasonic therapy (Lerner et al. 1973) as well as in ultrasonic diagnostics (Wells and Hills 1977), and on the international standardization for ultrasonic application in medicine (Ulrich 1974).

In a follow-up phase of the project (starting in 1984), two private German companies (Schoeller & Co., Moerfelden-Walldorf, and Buchler GmbH, Braunschweig) have committed themselves to the final development of the hardware and the introduction into clinical practice (planned for summer 1985).

Special Requirements and Restrictions of Ultrasonic Hyperthermia Equipment

The following points summarize the special requirements and limitations of therapeutic applicability of ultrasonic hyperthermia equipment, which have been used as a framework for its development.

1. A treatment volume of up to 50 ml located up to 8 cm below the surface is assumed to be typical.
2. The depth variation of the temperature maximum, including a periodic depth scan for smoothing out acoustic and thermal inhomogeneities, is considered indispensable.
3. A heat-up time of up to 5 min for a temperature increase from 37 °C to 42 °C–45 °C is considered desirable for clinical applications.

Recent Results in Cancer Research. Vol 101

4. Automatic invasive temperature control and monitoring with several thermocouples or thermistor elements has to be allowed until other noninvasive thermometry methods are available.
5. The possibility of simultaneous ultrasonic imaging of the therapy volume during treatment is desirable (noninvasive ultrasonic thermometry in the future seems feasible).
6. Operation frequency, acoustic power, and transducer geometry have to be optimized in order to achieve the desired temperature profile with a minimum of discomfort for the patient (heat and sound pressure peaks will eventually cause pain reactions and even tissue damage).
7. The design must take into account the physical limitations of ultrasonic application at tissue interfaces with extreme acoustic impedance differences (soft tissue/bone and soft tissue/lung) which result in overheating (bone) or insufficient penetration (lung); this automatically excludes certain treatment volumes.
8. Ultrasonic hyperthermia of body cavities (rectum, vagina, throat area) will require special applicators.

Approximation of Power Requirement

In an initial simplified approach we assume an isolated tissue volume of diameter D_T with heat capacity $\rho\, c_p$, where ρ is the tissue density. The required absorbed power $\dot{Q}_h$ for a heat-up time t_h then follows from:

$$\dot{Q}_h = \frac{\pi}{\sigma} D_T^3 \rho\, c_p \frac{\Delta T_{max}}{t_h} \tag{1}$$

When inserting typical values: $T_{max}=7$ K, $t_h=5$ min, $D_T=4$ cm, $c_p=3.8$ Ws/K cm^3, (muscle tissue) we find approximately 3 W to be necessary.

To keep this elevated temperature of the treatment volume stationary within a surrounding tissue of temperature T_0 and thermal conductivity k (typically $k=52\times10^{-4}$ W/K cm), the absorbed power required is:

$$Q_{st} = 2\,\pi\, D_T\, \Delta T_{max}\, k \tag{2}$$

with approximately 1 W in the above example. When thermal losses caused by perfusion are included (Lagendijk 1984), the required power increases by 0.5 W with normal perfusion (0.5 ml/kg) and by 5 W in the case of typical vasodilation (5 ml/kg). Therefore, the absorbed power required can be approximated to be 6 W.

Absorbed Acoustic Power

Figure 1 illustrates the radiation of acoustic energy from a circular disk transducer of diameter d_{tr} into a homogeneous, dissipative medium with absorption coefficient α. We assume near-field conditions (parallel sound beam) and ignore the near-field interference pattern, which is tolerable for long-term temperature considerations. In this case, the sound intensity I inside the sound beam can be assumed to be independent of the radial coordinate r and diminishes exponentially with increasing axial distance x from the transducer:

$$I(x) = I_0 \exp(-\alpha x) \tag{3}$$

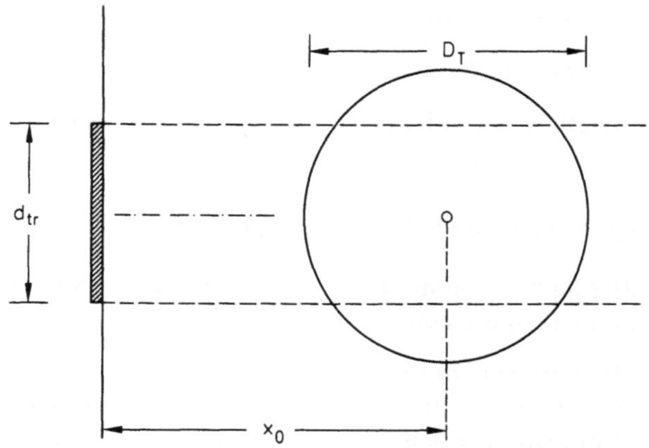

Fig. 1. Schematic illustration of tumor heating in the near field of a circular ultrasonic transducer. D_T, tumor diameter; d_{tr}, transducer diameter; x_0, distance between tumor center and surface

If the cylindrical sound beam penetrates a spherical partial volume with diameter $D_T > d_{tr}$, having a center distance x_0 from the surface of the dissipative medium, the absorbed power can be approximated by

$$\dot{Q}_{abs} = P_{rad}\alpha x_0 \exp(-\alpha x_0)\frac{D}{x} \leqq \frac{P_{rad}}{e}\frac{D}{x_0} \quad (4)$$

with P_{rad} being the acoustic power radiated by the transducer.

For a required absorbed power of 6 W with $D_T = 4$ cm and $x_0 = 5$ cm, a radiated acoustic power of roughly 20 W would then be necessary.

Optimization of Frequency

The acoustic power radiated into the dissipative medium is optimally utilized in the tumor volume (i.e., turned into heat) when the function

$$f(\alpha x_0) = \alpha x_0 \exp(1 - \alpha x_0) \quad (5)$$

is close to unity.

When tolerating a 20% efficiency loss [$f(\alpha x_0) \geqq 0.8$] compared with the maximum of Eq. (5), we find an optimal operation range

$$0.47 \leqq \alpha x_0 \leqq 1.8 \quad (6)$$

and since $\alpha \approx \alpha' f$ in biological tissue is almost a linear function of frequency, the optimal frequency range follows from

$$\frac{0.47}{\alpha' x_0} \leqq f \leqq \frac{1.8}{\alpha' x_0} \quad (7)$$

Introducing a typical absorption factor of muscle tissue ($\alpha' = 1$ dB/MHz cm) and a center depth of the tumor $x_0 = 5$ cm, the optimal frequency range

$$0.4 \text{ Mhz} \leqq f \leqq 1.6 \text{ Mhz}$$

would result.

Similarly we can select 1 MHz as typical frequency and find from Eq. (7)

$2\ \text{cm} \leqq x_0 \leqq 8\ \text{cm}$

as depth range with power utilization better than 80% of the available maximum.

Optimization of the Ultrasonic Applicator

After having optimized radiated power (20 W) and operation frequency (1 MHz), the remaining requirements had to be dealt with in the transducer design:

1. Heat maximum variable in depth ($2\ \text{cm} \leqq x_0 \leqq 8\ \text{cm}$)
2. Compatibility of treatment with simultaneous temperature monitoring (thermocouple)
3. Compatibility of applicator with simultaneous ultrasonic imaging
4. Power and temperature application with minimal discomfort for the patient (avoiding sound intensity and temperature peaks within the treatment area)

Fluid Lens Applicator with Variable Focal Length

Our first approach at an applicator for deep heating was designing a fluid lens with variable focal length, as shown in Fig. 2.

With a refractive index between Freon and water of $n = 2.7$ and the variable curvature of the spherically deformed plastic diaphragm, the focal length could easily be varied by hand between 2 cm and infinity (Fig. 2a). In a more sophisticated model (Fig. 2b), the focal length could even be varied automatically and periodically and, in addition, a motor-driven circumferential scanning of the focus was used to smoothen out the acoustic and thermal peaks in the focal zone by means of spatial-time averaging. Nevertheless, this approach turned out to be far from ideal.

Besides the incompatibility with simultaneous ultrasonic imaging and the intolerable offset reading of thermocouples in the intensive acoustic power range near the focus ($I < 100\ \text{W/cm}^2$)

$$\frac{\Delta T_{\text{offs.}}}{K} \approx 0.4 \frac{I}{W/\text{cm}^2} \frac{d^2}{\text{mm}^2} \tag{8}$$

(d is diameter of the thermocouple and I is sound intensity)

The single-focusing applicator was not able to focus heat into a volume area of a few milliliters in a long-term treatment. The thermal conduction spoiled the focussing effect for treatment lasting longer than a few minutes and on average the results were hardly different from those of treatment of nonfocussing flat transducers (Fig. 3). The main disadvantage, however, was the high acoustic power peak in the focal region, which resulted in intolerable pain reactions (animal experiments). Full-power focussing onto a cross section of less than 1 mm² (Fig. 4) was found impossible.

Small Cross Fire Applicator with Variable Focal Length

Our second design approach for an ultrasonic hyperthermia applicator is shown in Fig. 5. In this case, the well-known cross fire technique was used to compensate for acoustic absorption with increasing depth by the partially overlapping sound fields of six single

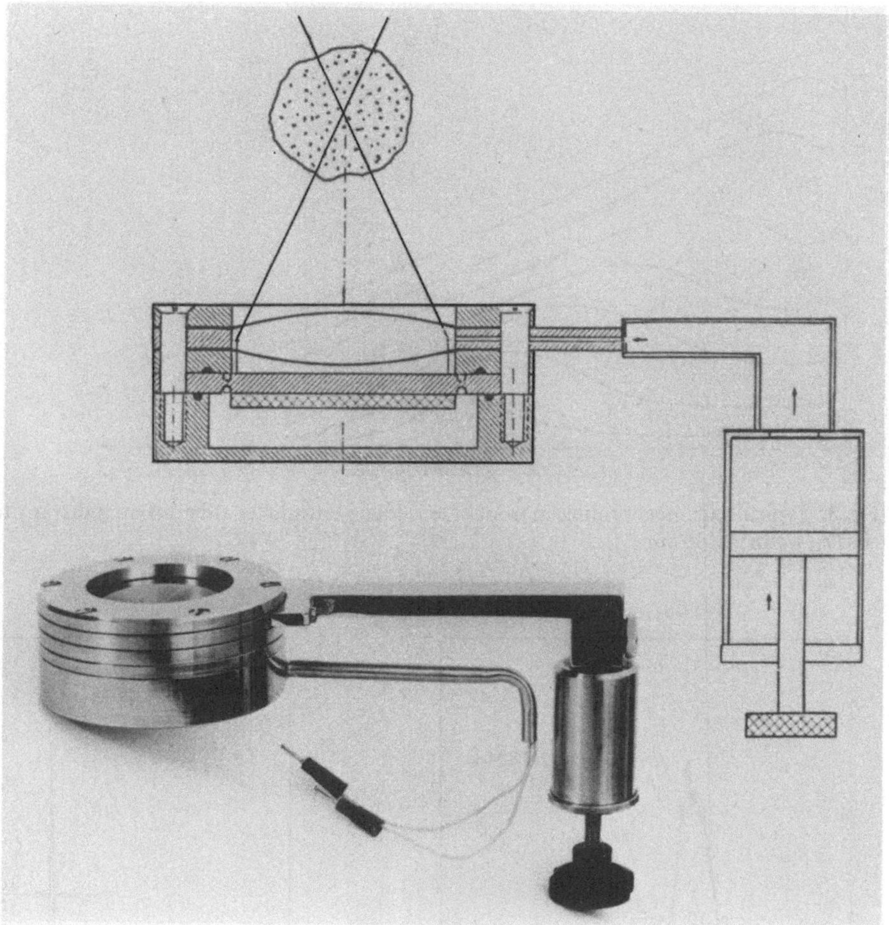

a

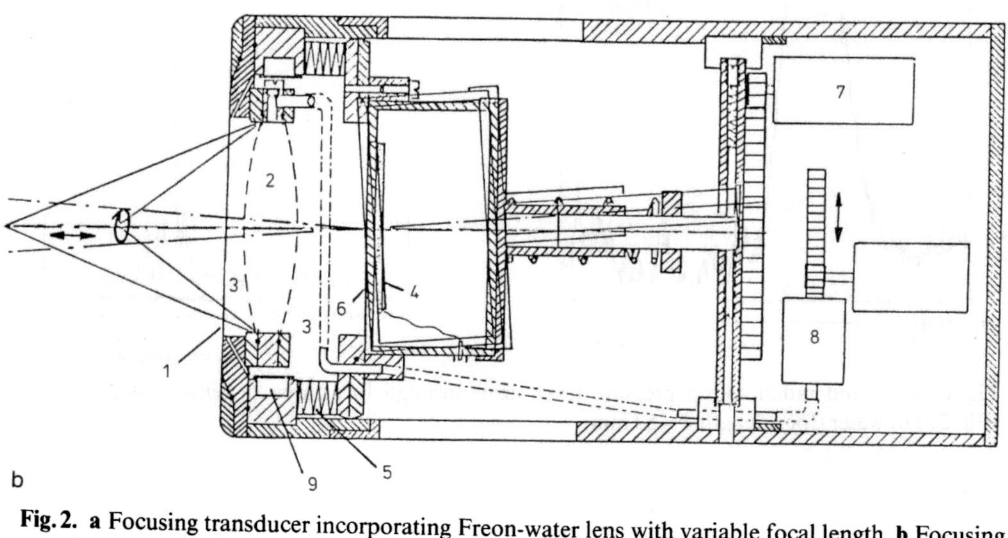

b

Fig. 2. **a** Focusing transducer incorporating Freon-water lens with variable focal length. **b** Focusing transducer as in **a** with automatic focal length variation (pump) and azimutal focus scanning (motor)

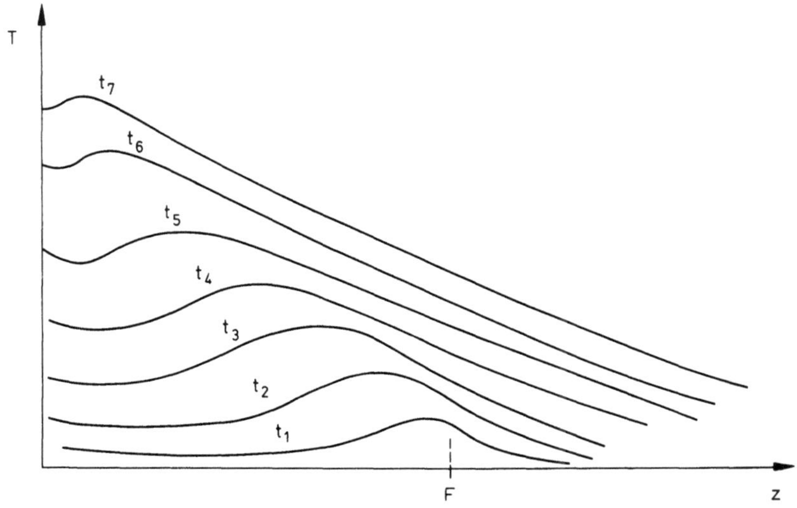

Fig. 3. Typical axial heat profiles in front of lens focus-transducer after different therapy times. *F*, focus; t_1, 1 min; t_5, 40 min

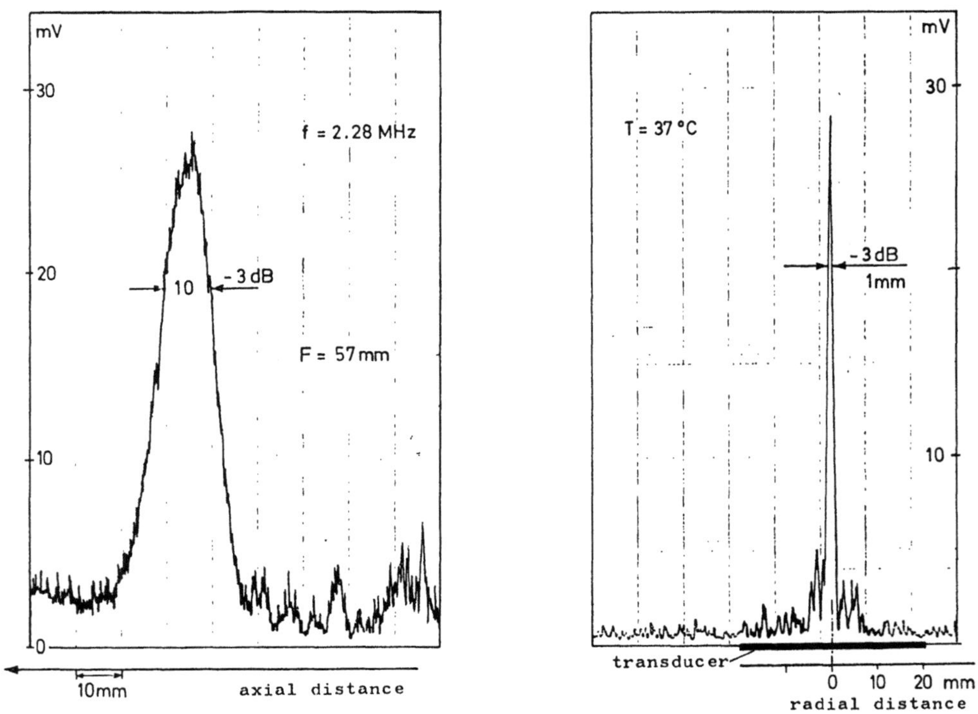

Fig. 4. Axial and radial sound pressure level scans through focal area of lens-focus transducer (Fig. 2a) in water (focal length $F=57$ mm)

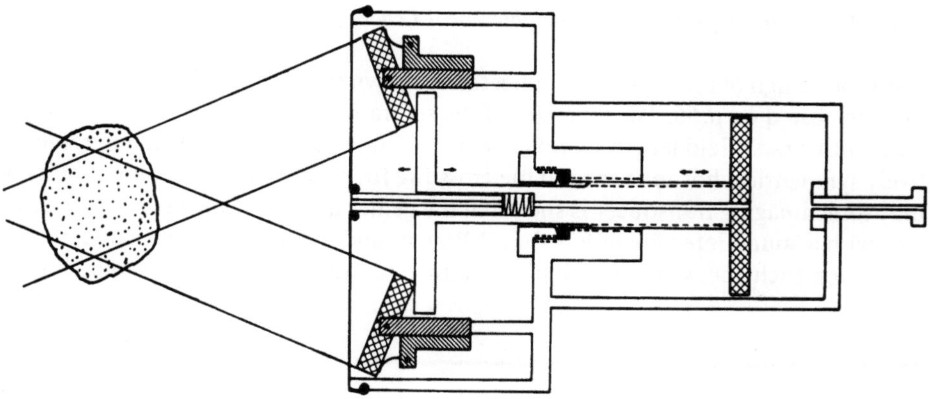

Fig. 5. Small cross fire applicator with six transducers (0.67 MHz, 15 mm effective diameter) and variable "focal length" (hand operated)

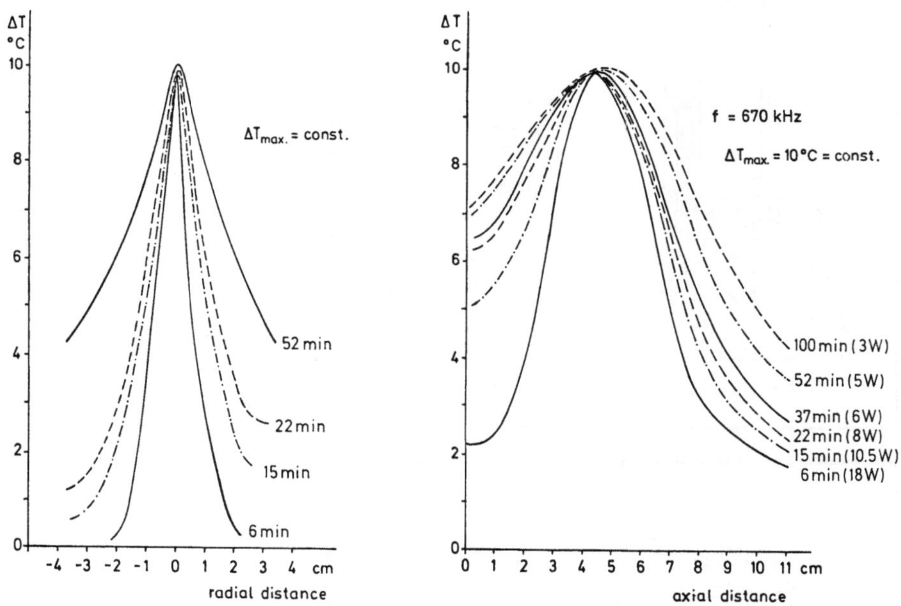

Fig. 6. Axial and radial temperature scans through focal area of cross fire applicator (cf. Fig. 5) in pork phantom. Power is adjusted to keep temperature peak constant at $\Delta T = 10\,°C$

transducers - each 15 mm in diameter - which radiate under the same - variable - angle against the common axis of the "array." The temperature distributions in the "focal range" measured in a tissue-mimicking phantom (Robrandt et al. 1981) with 1.2 dB/MHz cm absorption coefficient show good stability of the thermal focus within a desired therapy time of up to 2 h (Fig. 6).

The radial dimension of the hot zone, however, is small in comparison with the respective axial dimension. This is because the diameter of the transducer is too small.

Large Cross Fire Applicator with Variable Focal Length

The final design of the cross fire applicator as shown in Fig. 7 satisfied all the design specifications listed on p. 66. The diameter of the six transducers at 4 cm is large enough to operate with a near-field length (parallel beam) of more than 20 cm, which guarantees a relatively symmetrical hot zone around the cross fire focus (Fig. 8). Ideal compatibility with an ultrasonic imaging transducer is shown in the center of Fig. 7. Since each transducer radiates with a sound intensity of less than 1 W/cm^2 and the maximum radiated power is adjusted for each focus setting, highly irritating sound intensities are avoided and offset

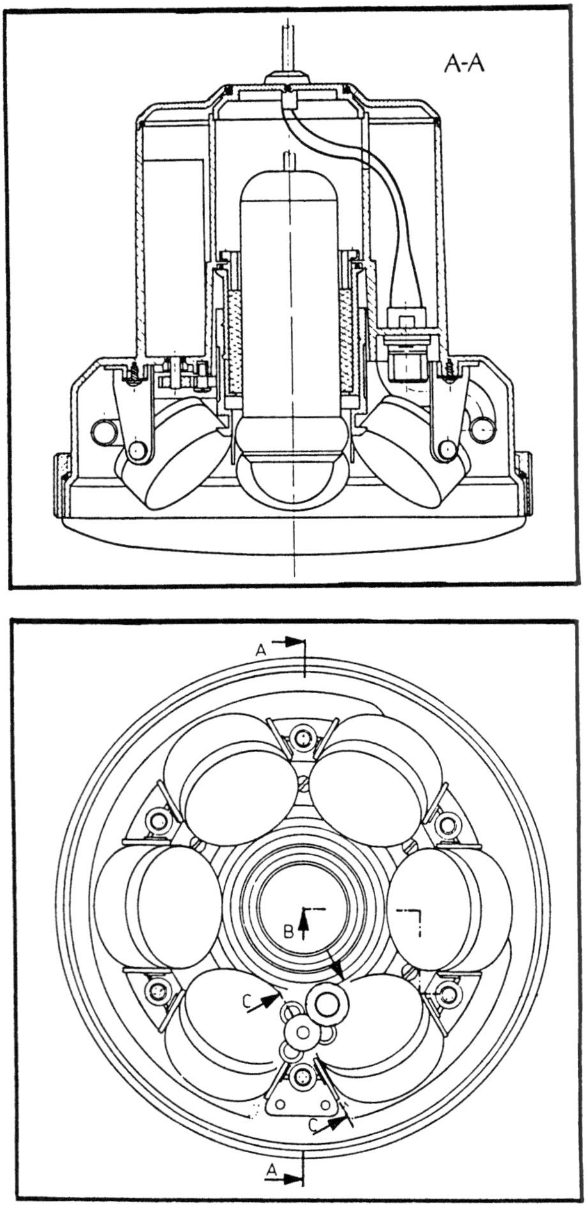

Fig. 7. Large cross fire applicator with six therapy transducers (1 MHz, 40 mm diameter) and diagnostic imaging transducer (*center*); "focal length" is variable (motor) between 2 and 8 cm in front of the diaphragm window of the thermostatized water-filled coupling section

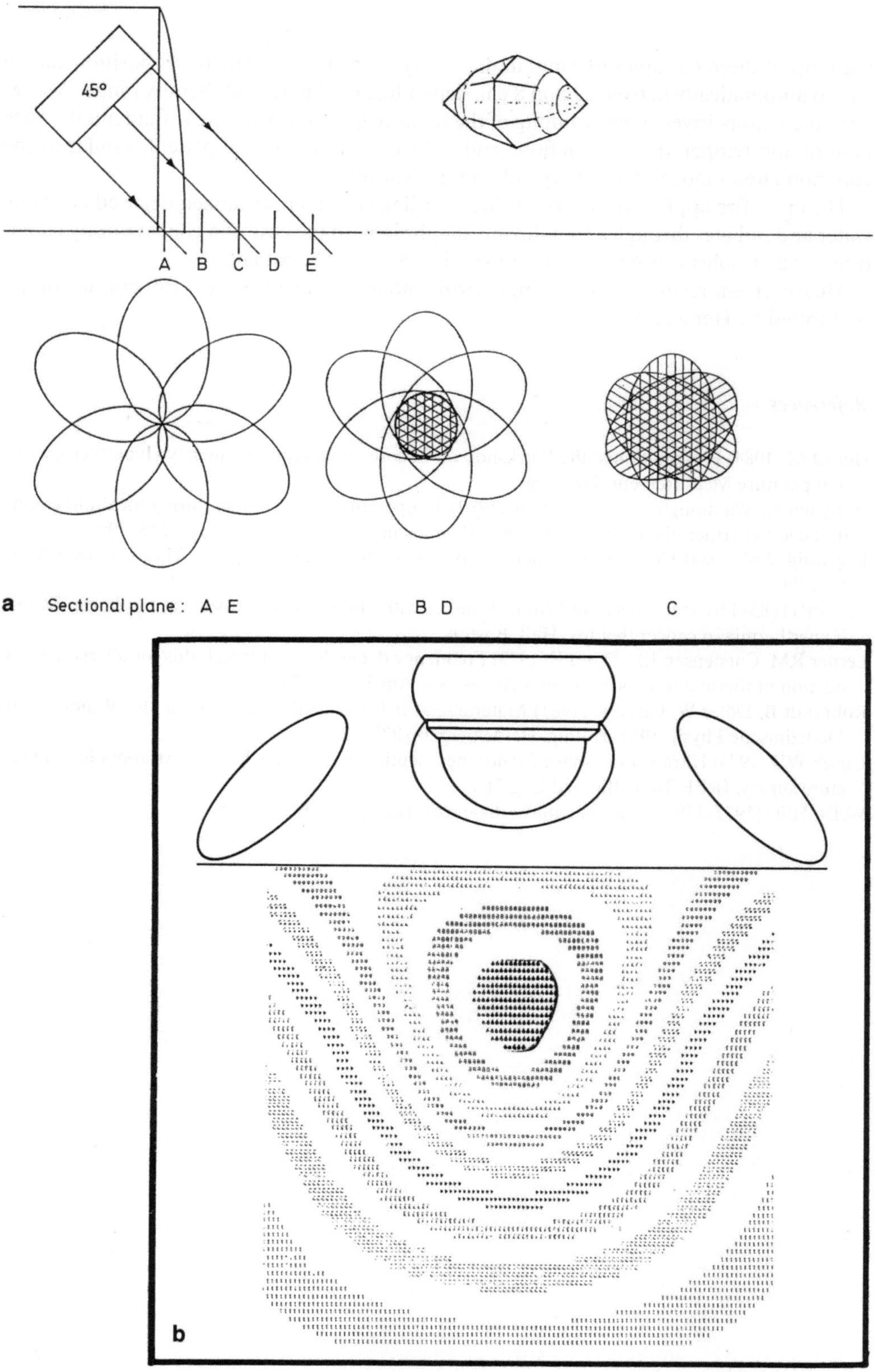

Fig. 8. a Typical overlapping sound beams (radial sections) in front of the cross fire applicator (cf. Fig. 7). **b** Calculated isotherms in homogeneous tissue in front of the cross fire applicator (Fig. 7)

readings of thermocouples (0.2 mm in diameter) are negligible. The focus position can be varied automatically between 2 and 8 cm, depending on the desired therapy range. A slow, periodic motor-driven axial scanning of the focus helps smooth out near-field interference pattern and temperature fluctuations and reduces irritation to the patient, similar to the common lateral movements of typical therapy transducers.

The cross fire applicator shown in Fig. 7 is filled with thermostatized degased coupling water and radiates through a thin flexible diaphragm. In the case of a concave body curvature, a water bolus is used as an additional interface to the patient.

Measurement results using the engineering model of the large cross fire applicator are performed by Herbst (1984).

References

Herbst M (1984) Presentation at the Workshop on Locoregional High Frequency Hyperthermia and Temperature Measurement, Freiburg

Hynynen K, Watmough DJ, Mallard JR (1982) Temperature distributions during local ultrasound induced hyperthermia in vivo. Ultrasonics Symposium. IEEE, New York, pp 745-799

Lagendijk JW (1984) Clinical hyperthermia: physical and technical aspects. Thesis, University of Utrecht

Lele PP (1983) Physical aspects and clinical studies with ultrasonic hyperthermia. In: Storm FK (ed) Hyperthermia in cancer therapy. Hall, Boston

Lerner RM, Carstensen EL, Dunn F (1973) Frequency dependence of thresholds for ultrasonic production of thermal lesions in tissue. J Acoust Soc Am 54: 504-506

Robrandt B, Döler W, Giese K (1981) Materialien für Ultraschall-Testphantome. In: Bunde E (ed) Medizinische Physik 1981. Hüthig, Heidelberg, pp 227-233

Ulrich WD (1974) Ultrasound dosage for nontherapeutic use of human beings, extrapolation of literature survey. IEEE Trans Biomed Eng 21

Wells, Hills (1977) Ultrasonics in clinical diagnosis. Livingston, Edinburgh

Thermometry and Thermal Modeling

Introduction

H. D. Kogelnik

Institut für Radiotherapie, Landeskrankenanstalten Salzburg, Müllner Hauptstrasse 48,
5020 Salzburg, Austria

Among the many centers using localized and regional hyperthermia in combination with ionizing radiation, there is general agreement about the clinical potential of this treatment method. There also seems to be general optimism about the clinical results obtained thus far.

However, there are problems associated with heating techniques including the calculation of a reliable thermal dosimetry, which is of utmost importance for the future of clinical hyperthermia. Temperature measurements remain a major problem, and currently there are no suitable noninvasive methods available.

We know from experimental in vivo data that - once the threshhold for tissue injury is reached - a small increase in hyperthermal treatment will cause a steep increase in the probability of tissue necrosis. Morris et al. (1977), for example, have shown that an increase of only 20% in heating time or less than 0.5 °C may increase the probability of tail necrosis in baby rats from 0% to 100%. It is therefore abvious that careful control of heat delivery and accurate thermometry are absolutely essential in clinical practice.

Furthermore, for a given level of reaction, it is important to know the relationship between temperature and treatment time. This relationship undergoes a transition between 42.5 °C and 43 °C. For temperatures above 43 °C, a change of 1 °C is equivalent to a change in heating time by a factor of 2. Below 42 °C the relationship alters and a change of 1 °C is approximately equivalent to a change in heating time by a factor of 6.

Within a localized treatment field, tumors may become hotter because of their more sluggish blood supply. However, the extent of any temperature differential that may occur will vary greatly from tumor to tumor. This is also true for any one patient with a given tumor during the 3- to 5-week course of multifractionated treatment.

Currently, thermometry for hyperthermia is based on invasive probes, which provide temperature measurements from a limited number of points. Because of the known biological responses, it is desirable to monitor and record temperatures with an accuracy of 0.1 °C.

Invasive probes for clinical practice should be smaller than 1 mm in diameter. For ultrasonic heating, very small thermistor and thermocouple probes are suitable. They pose problems, however, when used in electromagnetic fields. Specifically developed thermometers are now commercially available.

The positioning of a limited number of invasive probes within the tumor and the surrounding normal tissue is crucial for meaningful dosimetry in clinical hyperthermia. Through the work of Hand et al. (1982) we are aware of the significant temperature gra-

Recent Results in Cancer Research. Vol 101

dients which occur within the heated volume. The temperature-dependent tissue responses and the limiting maximum temperature in normal tissue also have to be considered. Therefore, monitoring temperature only in the assumed center of the tumor is quite unrealistic.

We all know that thermometry for clinical hyperthermia should be carried out by noninvasive methods. Several systems, based on nuclear magnetic resonance, microwaves, and ultrasound, are already under development.

References

Hand JW, Ledda JL, Evans NTS (1982) Temperature distribution in tissues subjected to local hyperthermia by RF induction heating. Br J Cancer [Suppl 5] 45: 31

Morris DD, Myers R, Field SB (1977) The response of the rat tail to hyperthermia. Br J Radiol 50: 576

Microwave Oncologic Hyperthermia Combined with Radiotherapy and Controlled by Microwave Radiometry

G. Giaux and M. Chivé

Centre de Lutte Contre le Cancer Oscar Lambret, BP 307, 59020 Lille Cédex,
Centre Médical Bourgogne, Rue de Bourgogne, 59000 Lille, France

In the group of high-frequency waves and electromagnetic radiation used in clinical hyperthermia, microwaves have a range of 434-2450 MHz. In the Proceedings of the Meeting held at Aarhus in 1984, it is mentioned that 983 evaluable lesions had been treated with microwave hyperthermia.

Since 1982, we have used microwave hyperthermia controlled by atraumatic radiometry to heat superficial tumors of a maximum thickness of 4 cm. This paper discusses the technical aspects and experimental observations of this type of hyperthermia, and the first clinical results of hyperthermia combined with radiotherapy are presented.

Technical and Experimental Studies

Microwave Hyperthermia Generators Controlled by Microwave Radiometry

Principle

Human tissues spontaneously emit electromagnetic radiation of thermal origin, which can be measured by a very sensitive receiver called a radiometer. When this measurement is carried out in the microwave frequency range where the tissues are relatively transparent, it is possible to evaluate the temperature of these tissues. This method constitutes a noninvasive technique of measuring the temperature of living tissues (Barret and Myers 1975; Carr et al. 1981; Mamouni et al. 1977).

Different microwave radiometers or microwave thermographs have been built in our laboratory and previous feasibility experiments have pointed out the possibility of achieving, in hyperthermia therapy, microwave local heating and microwave radiometry for temperature measurement with the same system (Nguyen et al. 1979, 1980).

Our system is characterized by the use of the same applicator for heating as well as for radiometric temperature measurement. In a typical radiometer, the amount of thermal noise power corresponding to a temperature variation of 1 °C is about 10^{-14} W. However, this system must radiate heating power in the order of a few watts. Thus to avoid any heating signals that reach the radiometer, it is necessary to have 150 dB isolation between the two branches of the system. According to this principle, our microwave system operates in an alternating mode: heat is applied at any time (switch in position 1), the temperature is

Recent Results in Cancer Research. Vol 101

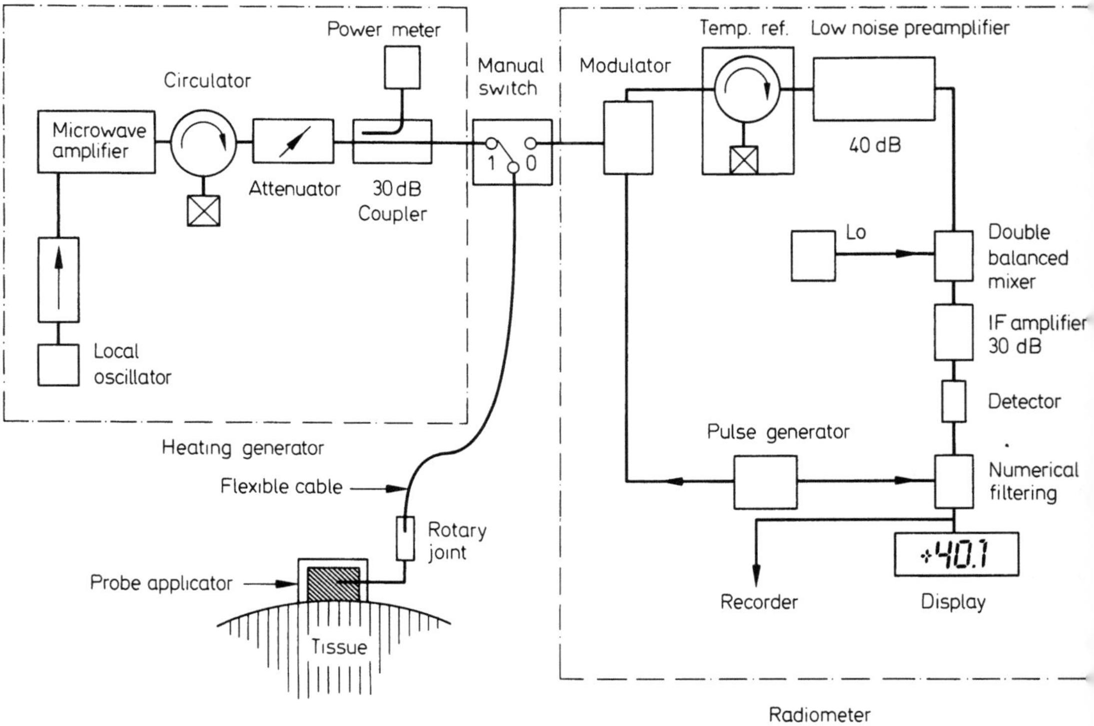

Fig. 1. Block diagram of the microwave hyperthermia system with temperature control by microwave radiometry

measured during the short intervals (for example, 5 s each minute) that the switch is in position 0 (Fig. 1) (Chivé et al. 1981; Nguyen et al. 1979, 1980).

To avoid any intermodulation from the generator to the radiometer, the heating generator is switched off during the radiometric temperature measurement.

Generators, Radiometers, and Applicators

Figure 1 shows the block diagram of the different prototype systems we have built according to the above principle. The microwave heating power is provided by a cavity oscillator followed by a microwave amplifier, which delivers an output power higher than 10 W at 2450 MHz and 130 W at 434 MHz.

Two microwave radiometers, which operate at around 3 and 1.2 GHz, respectively, with one GHz bandwidth around these central frequencies, have been associated with these generators. Each of them has the following characteristics: a measured noice factor of 5.5 dB and an experimental sensitivity of 0.2 °C (with a time constant of 2 s). Figure 2 gives the recorded radiometric signal versus time obtained with the 1-GHz radiometer when the applicator, isolated by a mylar sheet, is put on thermostated water, the temperature of which has been increased by about 1 °C at a definite time. Calibration of these radiometers is performed with water or a mixture of water and glycerol (30% glycerol + 70% water), which simulates biological tissues such as skin or muscle (Plancot 1983). A display allows direct reading of the measured temperature.

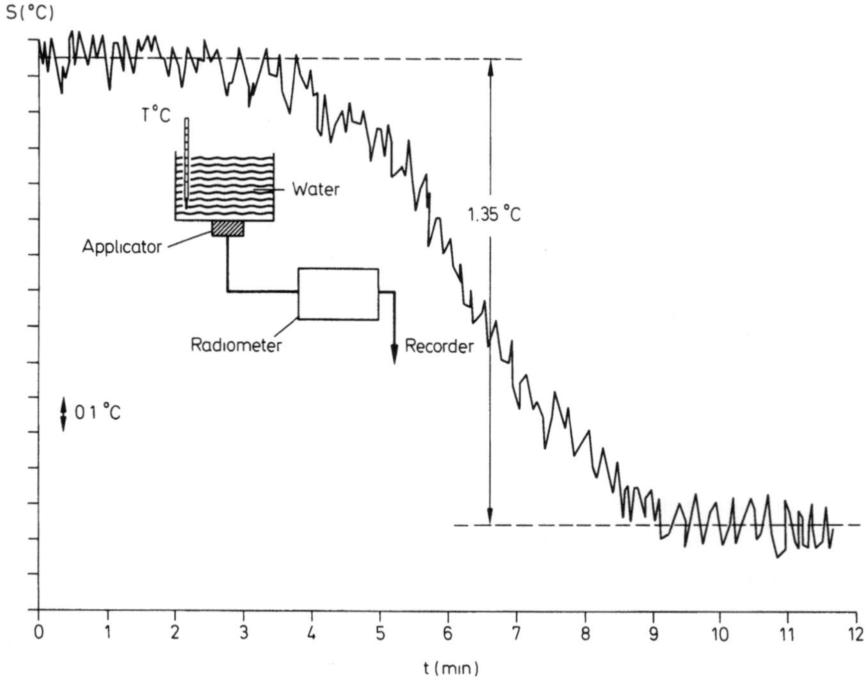

Fig. 2. Experimental sensitivity of the 1-GHz radiometer: recording of the radiometric temperature versus time

Two kinds of applicators have been used in these systems:

1. A rectangular waveguide filled with a low-loss solid dielectric ($\varepsilon_r = 25$) in order to reduce the dimensions of the aperture (6 × 3 cm here) and also to obtain a good match at the applicator tissue interface.
2. The second type of applicator we have developed is a microstrip-microslot antenna.

This probe applicator is designed by means of a gradual transition at constant impedance, from a classical microstrip line to a microstrip line with its ground plane opened. The applicator is formed by the ground plane aperture in contact with the tissue (Fig. 3) (Ringeisen et al. 1983). This type of applicator gives microwave performances higher than the waveguide type, as shown in Fig. 4, which shows the experimental measurements of the reflection coefficient (S_{11}) versus frequency for the two types of applicators put on a 90% water polyacrylamide gel (Plancot 1983), which simulates high water content tissue. Another feature of the microstrip-slot applicator is the possibility of central cooling by water flow in the cylinder put on the microstrip line in the aperture, as indicated in Fig. 3. This system avoids burns of superficial tissues during the heating session. These studies led to the development of the Hylcar I [Societé ODAM (office de diffusion d'appareillages médicaux), Wissembourg, France], an industrial system for clinical hyperthermia. It combines a 915-MHz microwave heating generator with a 2- to 4-GHz radiometer for temperature measurement and control and operates according to the alternate method, i. e., heat is applied at virtually any time and temperature is measured during short intervals.

In the Hylcar I, an interval-regulating circuit is inserted to control the balance between heating power and temperature measurement. The applicator used in the Hylcar system is a microstrip-microslot antenna which we have developed in our institute.

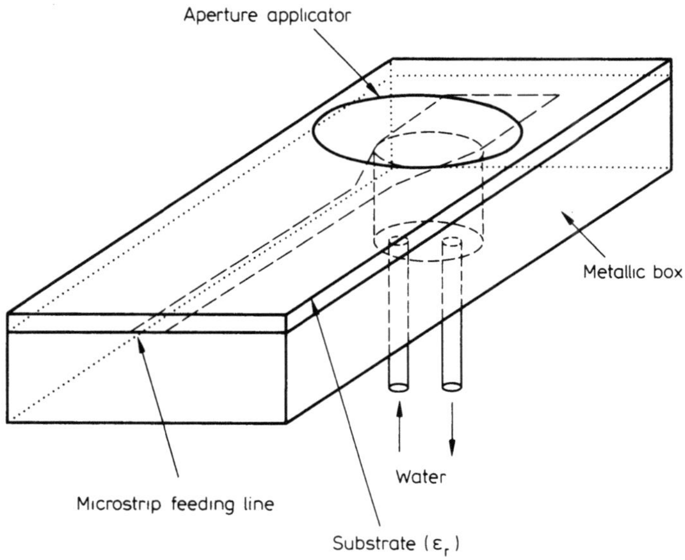

Fig. 3. Microstrip-microslot applicator with central cooling system

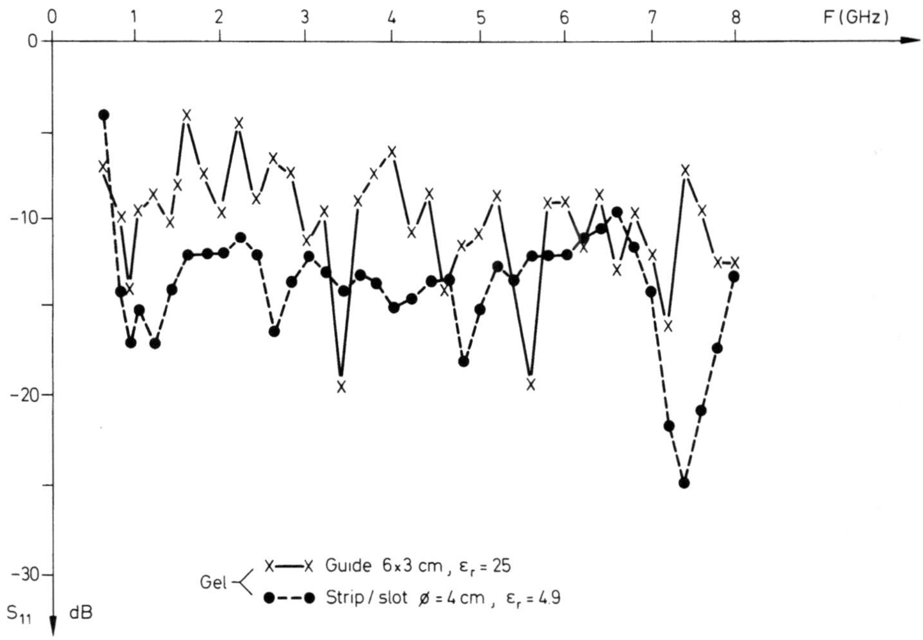

Fig. 4. Reflection coefficient S_{11} versus frequency measured on polyacrylamide gel for a guide (6×3 cm, $\varepsilon_r = 25$) and a strip-slot applicator ($\varnothing = 4$ cm, $\varepsilon_r = 4.9$)

Experiments

Numerous experiments on phantoms, excised tissues, and anesthetized animals were performed with these microwave systems before their application in hyperthermia therapy on patients (Chivé et al. 1982a, 1983a).

The biological phantom we used is a polyacrylamide gel in which a thermal gradient can be generated. Copper-constantan thermocouples (40 μV/°C) inserted at different depths measure the temperature inside the phantom in the heated zone under the probe applicator (Fig. 5). Isothermal profiles are then deduced from these measurements and compared with the radiometric temperatures. All of these temperature measurements are carried out when the heating generator is switched off. Figure 6 gives an example of isothermal profiles obtained in the phantom heated at 915 MHz by means of a microstrip-slot applicator with central water flow. The temperature measurement obtained with the 3-GHz radiometer is 44.2 °C, which corresponds to the temperature (measured by thermocouple) inside the phantom at 2.5 cm depth on the applicator axis. The 1-GHz radiometer gives a temperature measurement of 43 °C, which is the temperature at 3.5 cm on the axis of the probe. By means of the applicator the radiometers receive thermal signals produced by the lossy-heated phantom. Every subvolume of the medium radiates an isotropic thermal signal, which is proportional to its absolute temperature T and the radiometer bandwidth Δf (Rayleigh Jeans emission) but also depends on the dielectric properties of the lossy medium. Numerical calculations of the thermal noise signals emitted by homogeneous and multilayered lossy materials have been developed (Mamouni et al. 1977; Nguyen et al. 1979), particularly in the case of nonuniform temperature repartition, taking into account correlation and refractive-index variation effects. These computations show the influence of different parameters (frequency, temperature distribution, medium, etc.) on the radiometric temperature. Thus the two different experimental radiometric temperatures (Fig. 7) indicate that the investigated heated volume is deeper with the

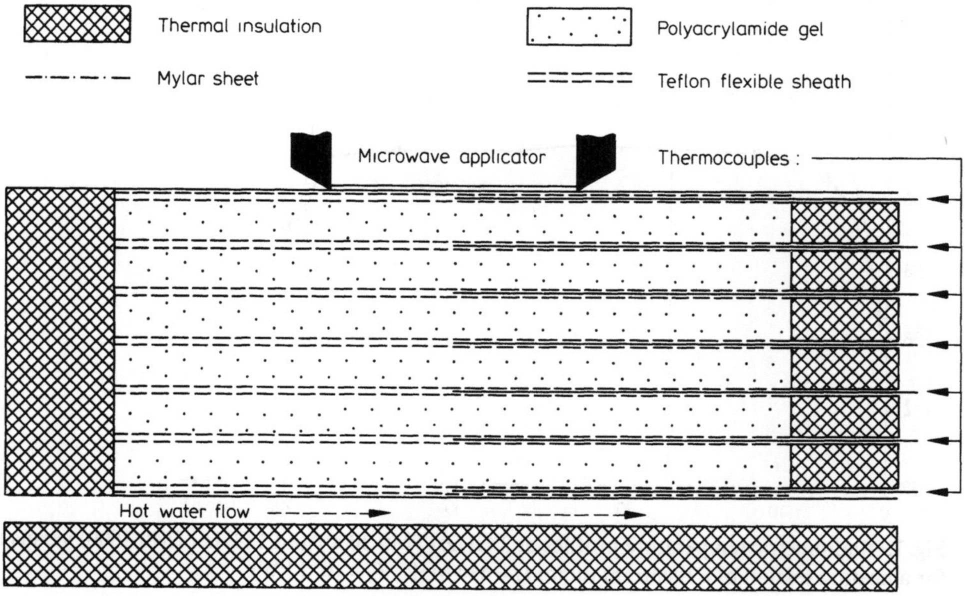

Fig. 5. Biological phantom with inserted thermocouples and hot water flow to generate initial thermal gradient

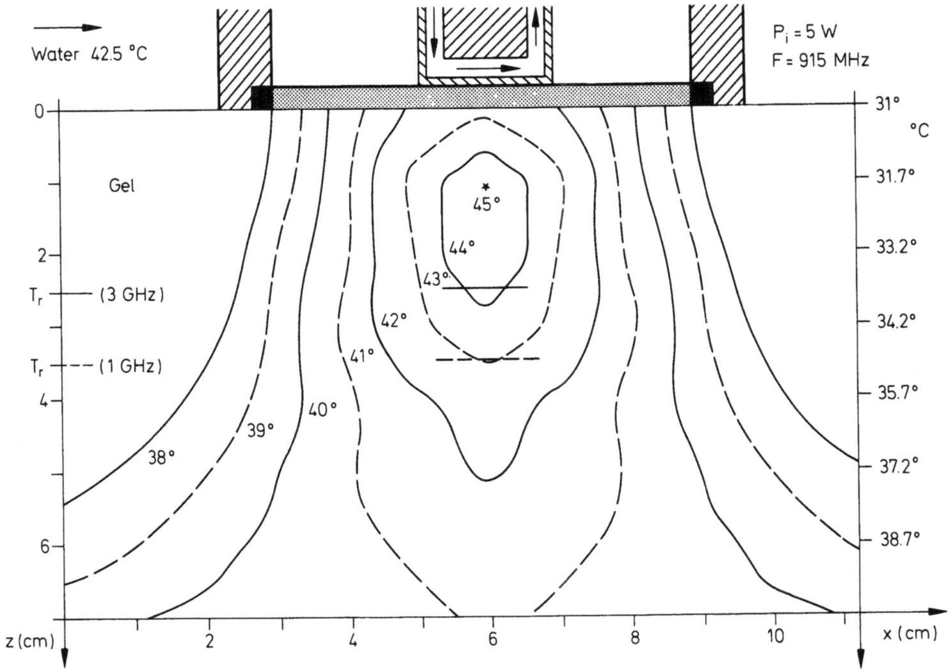

Fig. 6. Isothermal profiles in the phantom heated at 915 MHz ($P_i = 5$ W) with initial gradient (31°-38.7 °C) and central water flow (42.5 °C) in the applicator

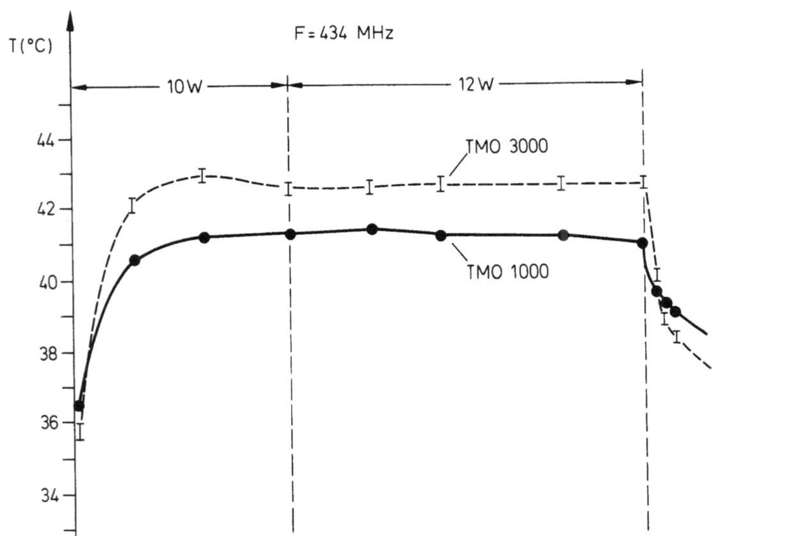

Fig. 7. Radiometric temperature profiles at 3 GHZ (TMO 3000) and 1 GHz (TMO 1000) versus time for a heating session of a recurrent tumor (f = 434 MHz, P_i = 10-12 W)

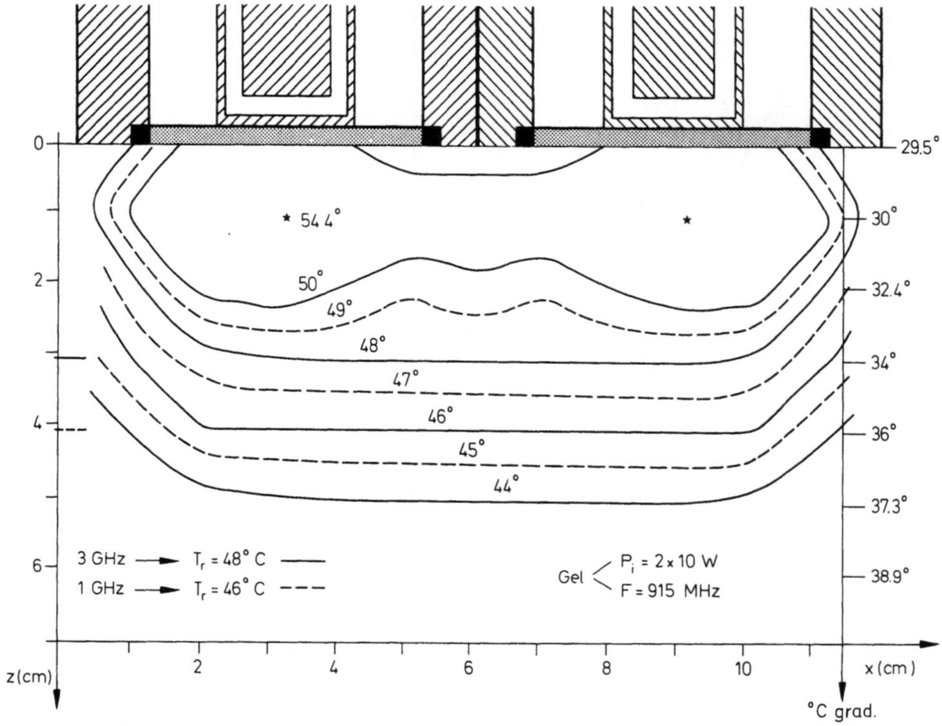

Fig. 8. Isothermal profiles obtained when the phantom (with an initial gradient) is heated with two identical applicators

1-GHz radiometer than with the 3-GHz radiometer. We can then say that the radiometric temperatures correspond to the "average temperature" of the heated volume coupled to the applicator in the bandwidth of the corresponding radiometer.

The use of two identical strip-slot applicators fed by the same incident power by means of a two-way in-phase power divider is illustrated in Fig. 8. It can be seen that the heated zone is larger and more uniform than that obtained with one applicator. The radiometric temperature measurements correspond to the temperature inside the phantom at 3 cm depth (for the 3-GHz radiometer) and 4-cm depth (for the 1 GHz radiometer).

Thermal Dosimetry in the Microwave Hyperthermia Process Based on Radiometric Temperature Measurements

Following the experiments on phantoms and the clinical treatments that we carried out in Lille, an atraumatic thermal dosimetry system was set up, which was based on the radiometric temperature measurements and the knowledge of the superficial temperature at the applicator-tissue interface during a heating session (Plancot 1983).

Two numerical programs have been developed to obtain the thermal profile on the axis of the applicator in the heated medium:

1. The first program calculates the thermal noise power emitted by homogeneous and multilayered lossy materials for a plane wave propagation, particularly in the case of a nonuniform temperature repartition.

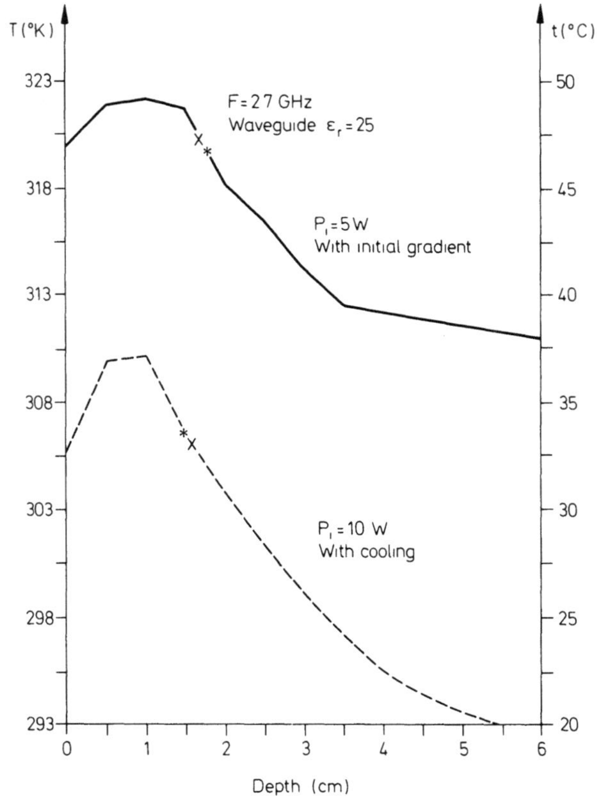

Fig. 9. Correlation between radiometric temperatures measured and calculated. *, measured temperature; ×, calculated temperature

2. The second computer program, based on the heat transport equation, calculates the thermal profile which occurs when the investigated medium is heated by a defined microwave power. From this calculated thermal profile, we can deduce the corresponding radiometric temperature by using the first program.

A numerical computer program taking into account the discontinuity at the applicator-tissue interface was set up to calculate the thermal noise power emerging from the investigated medium to the applicator. Figure 9 shows the good correlation between the theoretical and experimental radiometric temperatures during hyperthermia on a biological phantom (one case with an initial thermal gradient and another case in which the surface is cooled).

Numerical Simulation of Microwave Hyperthermia

A one-dimensional model was used, which defines the irradiated medium as a semiinfinite homogeneous layer. Taking into account superficial cooling and vascularization (in the case of tissue such as skin and muscle), the numerical program is based on the classical heat transport equation (Plancot 1983):

$$DC\,\frac{\delta T'}{\delta T} = Kt\,\frac{d^2\,T'}{dx^2} - V_S\,[T' - T_0] + Q'\,(x, t)$$

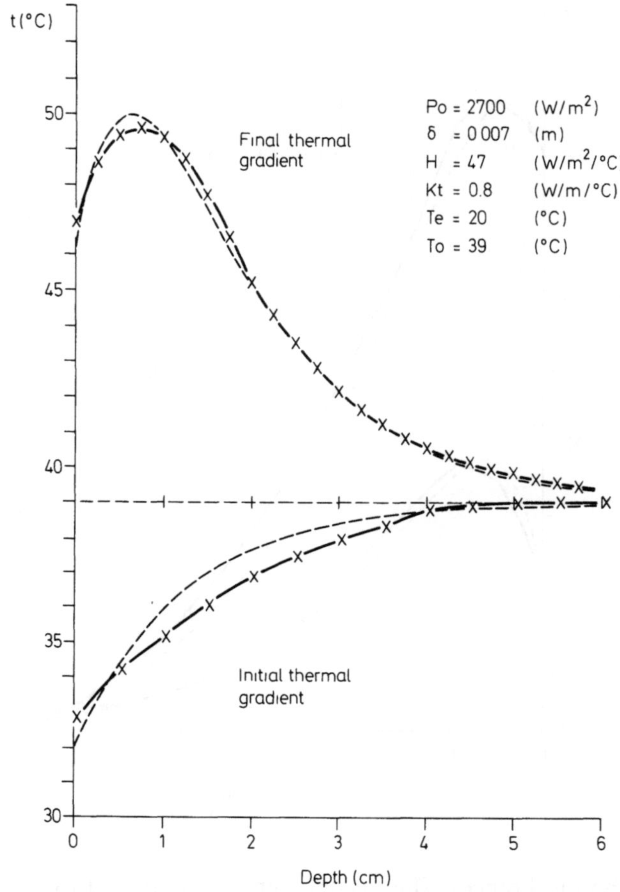

Fig. 10. Heat transport equation computation. × × ×, measured temperature; - - -, calculated temperature

where D = density of the medium, C = specific heat of tissue, K_t = thermal conductivity, V_s = heat exchange coefficent of blood, $Q'(x, t)$ = induced heat in tissue, $T'(x, t)$ = tissue temperature, and T_0 = blood temperature. This program used in the case of a microwave heating session on a biological phantom with initial gradient gives a thermal profile that correlates well with the experimental results (Fig. 10). Thus, using the first program it is then possible to calculate the radiometric temperature corresponding to this induced thermal profile.

From the experimental data, namely, the radiometric and superficial temperatures, the electrical and thermal characteristics of the medium, and the experimental conditions of microwave hyperthermia, we have calculated the thermal profile on the axis of the applicator by numerical computation using the two associated programs. With this inverse process we have obtained thermal gradients very close to those obtained in the experiment on the biological phantom (Fig. 11).

In conclusion, the method which now uses two different radiometric temperatures (around 1 GHz and 3 GHz) to obtain more information and precision in the determination of the thermal profile in tissue can be extended to achieve atraumatic thermal dosimetry in the hyperthermia process for cancer treatment on patients.

Based on these technical and experimental studies, a new industrial apparatus for clinical hyperthermia has recently been designed: the Hylcar II (Society ODAM, Wissem-

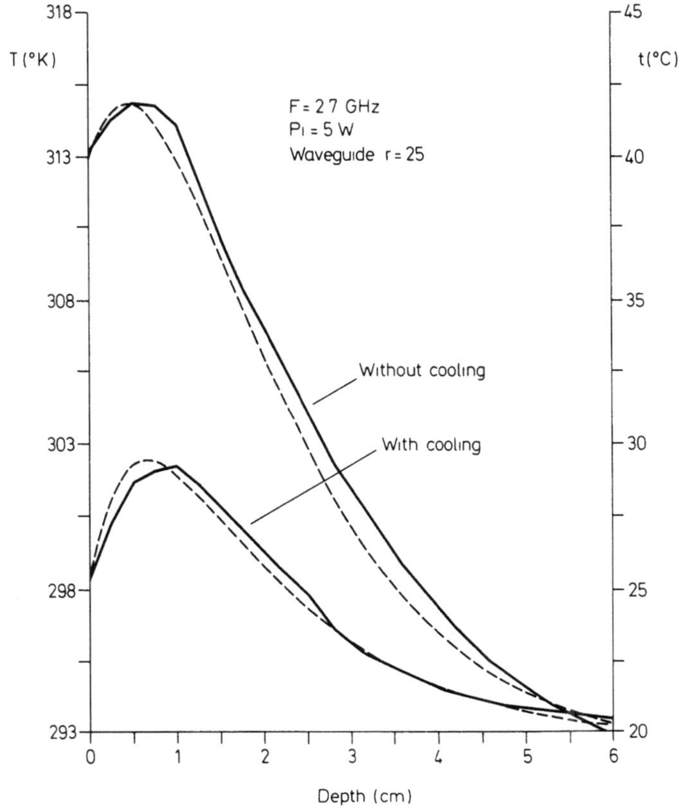

Fig. 11. Comparison between theory and experiments. —, measured gradient; - - -, computed gradient

bourg, France). This second-generation apparatus associates two heating generators of 915 and 2450 MHz, with two radiometers working in the bands 0.8–2 and 2–4 GHz, and is monitored by a computer.

The study of the feasibility and of the therapeutic advantages of this apparatus has been initiated by a hyperthermia study group as part of a program: the *TEP* procedure (*Transfert et Evaluation de Prototype,* French State Departments of Health and Research).

Clinical Studies

Local microwave hyperthermia was applied for the treatment of superficial primary or recurrent tumors of a thickness up to 3–4 cm. These tumors account for about 35% of all tumors treated by radiotherapy with electrons.

Patients and Methods

We used 0.434-, 0.915-, and 2.4-GHz generators and studied the feasibility of a prototype 915 MHz (Hylcar I, ODAM Society, Wissembourg, France).

Heating was carried out on phantoms made with methylacrylamide gel, which have dielectric characteristics nearly similar those of the muscle. Measurements were also made on anesthetized animals.

In experimental and clinical studies, temperature measurements were carried out with a radiometric receiver working in 0.8- to 2- and 2- to 4-GHz bands and thermocouples with a good correlation. We used waveguides and, later, microstrip-microslot applicators with a cooling system inserted. Using two or four applicators working in phase, it is possible to increase the size of the treated volumes and to homogenize the temperatures (Chivé et al. 1983b).

Phases I and II of the clinical trials dealt with superficial carcinoma with a maximum thickness of 4 cm. Treatment was carried out on primary advanced tumors and recurrent tumors in previously irradiated areas or that had been treated by radiotherapy and surgery. The same applicators were used for heating and for the temperature measurements. The two functions alternatively used provided an atraumatically controlled treatment. The surface of the applicator, which was applied on the tumor site, was maintained at the desired temperature by regulating the temperature of the water inside the probe.

The main protocols applied were (Giaux et al. 1983, 1984):

1. Combination with external radiotherapy with electrons and brachytherapy.
   Radiotherapy: two sessions a week, applying 4 Gy at each session. The total dose is 30-35 Gy for recurrent tumors and 50-65 Gy for primary tumors. The sessions are immediately followed by hyperthermia application for a period of 1 h. After the end of radiotherapy, hyperthermia is continued alone for up to 15-20 sessions.
   Contact X-ray radiotherapy: the same protocol as above, or three or four sessions of 15-20 Gy. Hyperthermia is carried out 1 h after the irradiation.
   In brachytherapy, local hyperthermia is applied for 1 h immediately before and after the application with radioactive sources.
2. Combination with chemotherapy: local hyperthermia is performed during the perfusion of the drugs.

Results

In a period of 28 months, we carried out more than 1070 microwave hyperthermia sessions on 70 patients. Hyperthermia was combined with external radiotherapy, brachytherapy, or chemotherapy, or applied alone after the end of radiotherapy. We recorded 25 first-degree burns, which healed in 10 days, and 5 local second-degree burns, which healed in 4-6 weeks.

Forty-seven lesions have been followed-up between 3 and 20 months after the end of the treatment:

Thirteen primary advanced and inoperable tumors - one melanoma of the eyelid, three squamous-cell carcinomas of the eyelid, two squamous-cell carcinomas of the nose, one cutaneous metastasis of a melanoma, one inoperable vaginal carcinoma, two inoperable breast neoplasms, one large and infiltrating carcinoma of the skin of the forehead, and two rectal carcinomas. Ten of these lesions are in complete regression and three showed partial regression. Two of these partial regressions are advanced rectal localizations, for which surgical treatment was not possible. The other was a lesion of the inferior half of the nose with extension to the cartilage; the patient was a 95-year-old woman whose general condition has not enabled regular treatment to be carried out.

There were 34 recurrences in previously irradiated areas: 16 cervical or supraclavicular nodes, 11 chest-wall cutaneous recurrences of breast carcinoma, 1 carcinoma on a scar of an old burn, 2 cutaneous carcinomas of the cheek, 3 extensions of buccal carcinoma, and

1 pyriform sinus carcinoma. Twenty-eight of these lesions are in complete regression. A partial regression was observed for the six other localizations.

Discussion

Tolerable surface temperature conditions are as follows:

1. For one applicator: 42° -43 °C at a depth of 3 cm with a useful surface of 4.5-25 cm^2
2. For two applicators: 42° -43 °C at a depth of 4 cm with a useful surface of 14-60 cm^2
3. At 434 MHz and with four applicators we can heat a surface of 140 cm^2

In practice, the temperature of the deeper part of the tumor must be maintained between 42° and 43 °C (+/− 0.5 °C). The possibility of thermotolerance reactions made us decide on a 72-h interval between hyperthermia sessions.

If the radiotherapy can be essentially concentrated on the lesions, irradiation sessions are immediately followed by hyperthermia. If the radiotherapy can affect an important peritumoral healthy tissue volume, we suggest an interval of 4 h between irradiation and hyperthermia.

Other authors have also obtained encouraging results with microwave hyperthermia (HT) applied with radiotherapy (RT).

Some reports of comparative clinical trials include:

1. Lindholm et al. (1984): lesions treated by RT alone, 28% complete regression; RT and HT, 39% complete regression.
2. Scott et al. (1983) report the therapeutic results observed in patients with at least two lesions, one being treated by RT alone and one other with the combination of RT and HT. The results of the latter type of treatment were always better for the different protocols studied (Radiotherapy Treatment Oncology Group, RTOG).
3. Arcangeli and Nervi (1984) studied phase III trials with different protocols. For each of them they found an increase in the therapeutic gain factors (TGF) when microwave hyperthermia was combined with RT.

Indeed, the numbers of patients reported on are relatively small; however, all of the publications confirmed the therapeutic advantage of the combination of microwave hyperthermia and radiotherapy versus radiotherapy alone.

From these results different types of clinical trials with microwave hyperthermia of phase II and III are being planned (by the RTOG, among others). A French group is planning the *TEP* procedure (TEP=transfert evaluation de prototype) for the State Departments of Health and Research.

Conclusion

During local microwave hyperthermia, atraumatic temperature control is a factor of safety and efficiency. The use of microstrip-microslot applicators enables accurate adjustment to individual cases to be made. Microwave hyperthermia seems to be an efficient complementary method of treating superficial tumoral carcinomas up to 3-4 cm in depth, primary tumors, or recurrences in previously irradiated areas. Nevertheless, clinical hyperthermia, even with microwaves, must be applied with great care. But the results published during the past few years are an encouragement to continue to develop a complementary method which can improve the treatment of cancer.

References

Arcangeli G, Nervi C (1984) The clinical use of experimental parameters to evaluate the response to combined heat (HT) and radiation (RT). Proceedings of the 4th International Symposium on Hyperthermic Oncology, Aarhus, Denmark, pp 329-332

Barret AH, Myers PC (1975) A method of detecting subsurface thermal patterns. Biol Radiol 6: 45-56

Carr KL, El Madhi AM, Schaffer J (1981) Dual mode microwave system to enhance early detection of cancer. IEEE Trans Microwave Theory Tech 29: 256-260

Chivé M, Leroy Y, Giaux G, Prévost B (1981) Microwave thermography for controlled local hyperthermia at 2.5 GHz. Digest of the 16th Microwave Power Symposium, Toronto

Chivé M, Plancot M, Leroy Y, Giaux G, Prévost B (1982a) Process in microwave and radiofrequency hyperthermia controlled by microwave thermography. 3rd International Congress of Thermology, Bath, England

Chivé M, Plancot M, Leroy Y, Giaux G, Prévost B (1982b) Microwave (1 and 2.45 GHz) and radiofrequency (13.56 MHz) hyperthermia monitored by microwave thermography. 12th European Microwave Conference Proceedings, Helsinki

Chivé M, Plancot M, Leroy Y, Giaux G, Prévost B (1983a) Microwave hyperthermia monitored by microwave thermography: technical aspects and clinical results. 18th Microwave Power Symposium Proceedings, Philadelphia

Chivé M, Plancot M, Giaux G, Prévost B, Delannoy J (1983b) Technical aspects of microwave hyperthermia monitored by microwave thermography. Strahlentherapie 159: 369

Chivé M, Plancot M, Vandevelde JC (1983c) Wide band microstrip-slot applicators for microwave hyperthermia and microwave thermography. 18th Microwave Power Symposium Proceedings, Philadelphia

Fabre JJ, Leroy Y (1981) Thermal noise emission of a lossy material for a TEM propagation. Electron Lett 17

Giaux G, Prévost B, Delannoy J, Chivé M, Plancot M (1983) Microwave hyperthermia associated with radiotherapy and atraumatic control by microwave thermometry: first clinical observations. Strahlentherapie 159: 372-373

Giaux G, Prévost B, Delannoy J, Chivé M, Plancot M (1984) Local microwave hyperthermia combined with radiotherapy in the treatment of cancer: clinical results. Proceedings of the 4th International Symposium on Hyperthermic Oncology, Aarhus, Denmark, pp 338-340

Lindholm CE, Kjellen E, Landberg T, et al. (1984) Microwave-induced hyperthermia and radiotherapy. Clinical results. Proceedings of the 4th International Symposium on Hyperthermic Oncology, Aarhus, Denmark, pp 341-344

Mamouni A, Bliot F, Leroy Y, Moschetto Y (1977) A modified radiometer for temperature and microwave properties measurements of biological substances. Proceedings of the 7th European Microwave Conference, Copenhagen, p 703

Nguyen DD, Mamouni A, Leroy Y, Constant E (1979) Simultaneous microwave local heating and microwave thermography. Possible clinical applications. J Microwave Power 14 (2)

Nguyen DD, Chivé M, Leroy Y, Constant E (1980) Combination of local heating and radiometry by microwaves. IEEE Trans Instrum Meas 29: 143-144

Plancot M (1983) Contribution à l'étude théorique, expérimentale et clinique de l'hyperthermie microonde contrôlée par radiométrie microonde. Thesis, University of Sciences and Techniques, Lille

Ringeisen V, Chivé M, Toutain S (1983) Applikator zum Zu- oder Abführen von Hochfrequenzenergie. Applicator for supplying energy to and from an object. Patent, n° P33006776, Federal Republic of Germany

Robillard M, Chivé M, Leroy Y (1981) Toward an interpretation of the thermal signatures achieved by microwave thermography. Digest of the 16th Microwave Power Symposium, Toronto

Scott RS, Johnson RJR, Kowal H, et al. (1983) Hyperthermia in combination with radiotherapy: a review of five years experience in the treatment of superficial tumors. Int J Radiat Oncol Biol Phys 9: 1327-1333

The Applicability of Microwave Thermography for Deep-Seated Volumes

G. Bruggmoser and W. Hinkelbein

Universitätsklinik, Abteilung für Röntgen- und Strahlentherapie im Zentrum Radiologie, Hugstetter Strasse 55, 7800 Freiburg i. Brsg., FRG

Introduction

The clinical application of hyperthermia as an additional modality to radiotherapy or chemotherapy requires a knowledge of the temperature distribution throughout the region to be treated (Divrik et al. 1984).

According to in vitro studies performed by Dewey et al. (1977), temperature differences of just a few tenths of a degree can affect the results considerably. Such precise measurement, especially in a deep-seated region, is hardly possible. However, the necessity for several reproducible treatment sessions requires adequate thermometry in order to regulate a microwave unit.

Requirements of a Clinical Thermometry System

Hand (1984) and Christensen (1983) proposed some factors required by a thermometry system. The temperature range from 20 °C to 55 °C should be measured with an accuracy and resolution of 0.1 °C. A spatial resolution of about 1 cm is desirable and the response time should be within 1 s. An important factor is the long-term stability of the thermometry system. During at least one treatment period, the system should work without additional calibration.

One group of thermometer probes includes thermocouples, thermistors, and crystals connected to fibers (Christensen 1983; Vaguine et al. 1984). These are used as invasive probes. One problem with these probes is puncturing with hollow needles at each treatment session in order to insert multiple probes into the tissue. This method can be applied in regions close to the surface. An alternative for treatment of deep-seated regions is to implant probes which will remain in the tissue during all of the treatment sessions. The two main problems of these procedures are: (1) the additional strain of the patient caused by the surgical implantation and (2) the technical problem of interference, especially of the metallic probes and leads with the electromagnetic field (Bliek and Heizmann 1976; Nilsson 1984). For these reasons several groups are working on the development of further thermometry systems which will fulfill the physical as well as the clinical conditions.

Recent Results in Cancer Research. Vol 101

Microwave Thermometry

Another possible thermometry method is microwave thermometry, which is a noninvasive method. Microwave thermometry entails the recording of radiation emitted from the body in a wavelength of between 1 mm and 1 m. The correlation between the received radiation of the antenna and the emitted radiation from the tissue is given by the Nyquist formula: The exchange radiation power is proportional to the object temperature T_0 and the bandwidth B:

$$P = T_0 B k \tag{1}$$

where k = the Boltzmann constant.

The advantage of microwave thermography would be that the same antenna could be used for both the microwave generator and for the receiver. This means that within one hyperthermia treatment session the fixation of the applicators is identical to the fixation of the thermometry unit.

The development of microwave radiography systems has been in progress for several years. Well-known publications include those by the group at the University of Lille (Nguyen et al. 1980; Plancot 1983; Plancot et al. 1984), the Philips Laboratory in Hamburg (Lüdeke 1983), and several institutions in the United States (Porter and Miller 1978). Among these groups, those of the Massachusetts Institute of Technology (MIT) (Myers et al. 1979) and the University of Denver are particularly well known (Edrich 1984).

Our subject is the heating of deep-seated lesions. Therefore, it is necessary to obtain

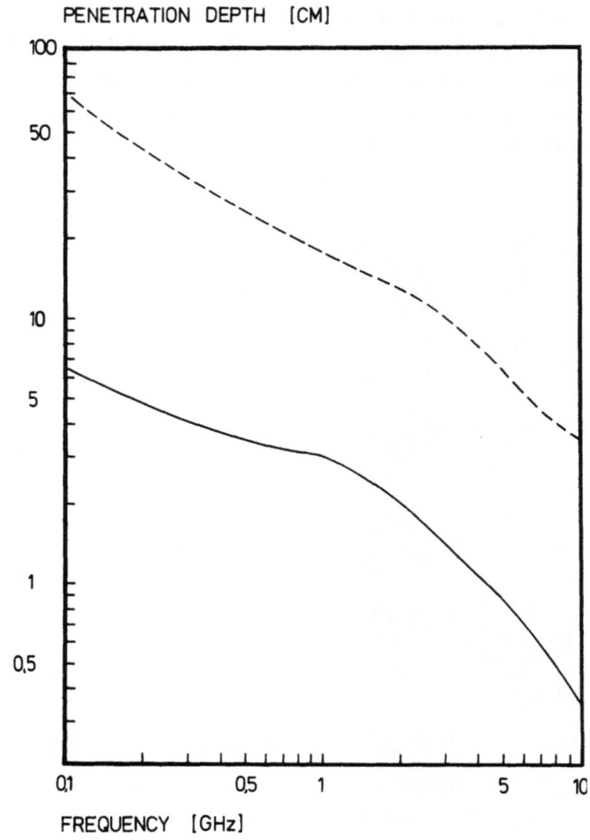

Fig. 1. Frequency-dependent penetration depth of electromagnetic radiation into tissue. - - -, dry tissue: bone, fat; ——, wet tissue: skin, muscle

some information on the temperature distribution in this region. That is why we try to apply microwave thermography in a frequency range around 300 MHz (Fig. 1). As can be seen from Fig. 1, the depth of penetration of microwaves in tissue depends on their frequency; the lower the frequency the better the penetration depth. In terms of the microwave radiation emitted from the tissue, there is a better chance of a signal being given off from the deeper regions (NCRP 1981).

Material

The measurements presented were performed with a prototype of a hyperthermia system developed by Bruker/Odam, Rue d'Industrie, Wissembourg. This system consists of two microwave generators with a frequency of 434 MHz and a microwave receiver operating in the frequency band of about 100–500 MHz (Fig. 2). The two generators work in the master and slave system, that is, one generator is connected to the thermography unit which controls the microwave power. The system works with several contact applicators; one of them is designed to transmit and to receive. The sequence of microwave power and measurement can be switched from 1 to 5 min emitting, and 12 s receiving. The result of the temperature measurement is compared with the chosen temperature and effects a decrease or increase in the power of the generators. According to Plank's law (Gerthsen and Kneser 1969), calculated with a human body core temperature of 310 K, the energy density of the radiation around 300 MHz is about 10 powers lower than that of infrared (Fig. 3). An additional problem is radio and TV stations in the 100-MHz frequency range. From our first measurement we learned that without a Faraday cage there is no way of obtaining reliable results (Fig. 4).

All experiments should include an initial check of the suitability of the system. To obtain standard conditions, these experiments were performed with only one applicator, working in the emitting and receiving mode. In this context, we examined the applicability of the system and not the technical details of the unit.

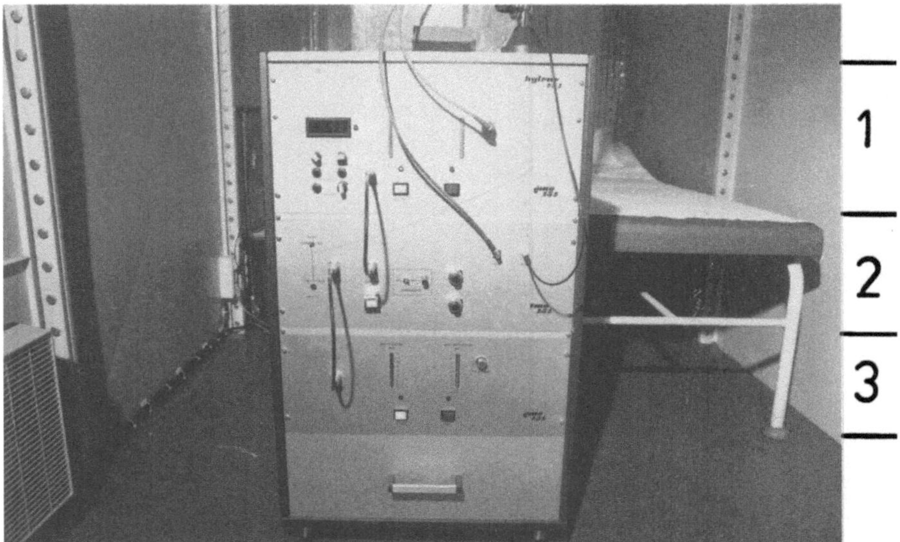

Fig. 2. Hyperthermia system built by Bruker/Odam. *1+3*, microwave generator, 434 MHz; *2*, microwave receiver operating in the frequency band of 100–500 MHz

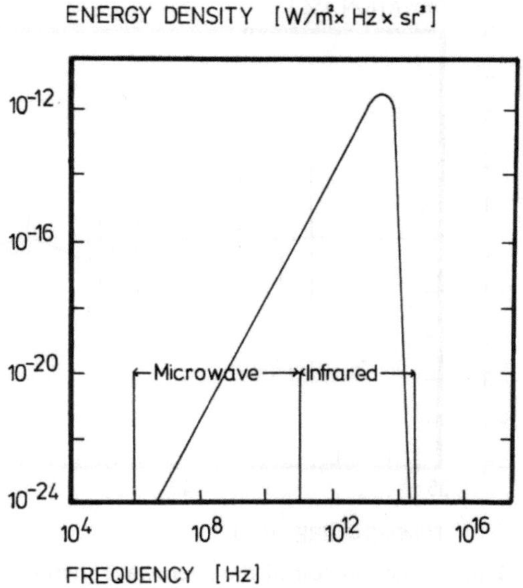

Fig. 3. Planks law: frequency-dependent energy density, calculated with a core temperature of the human body of 310 K

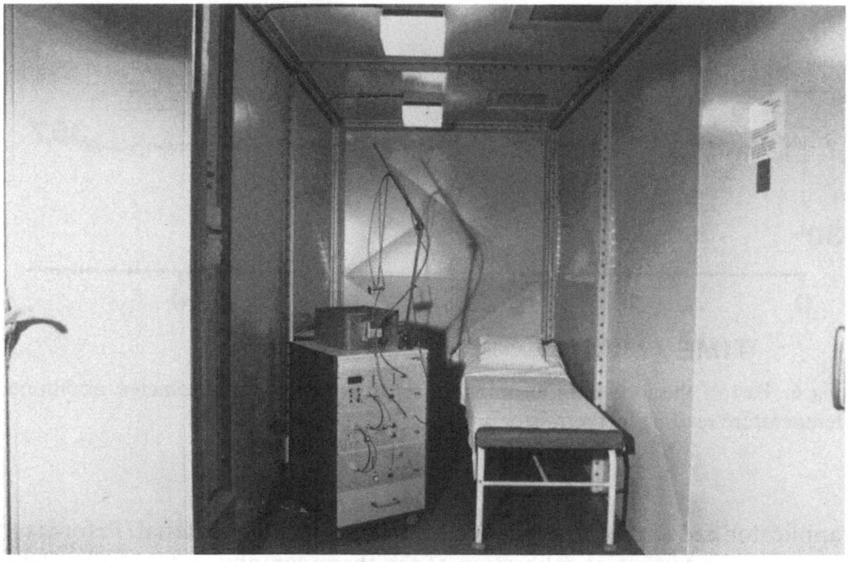

Fig. 4. Treatment unit consisting of a Faraday cage and the hyperthermia system

Experiments with a Homogeneously Heated Volume

Range, Accuracy, and Resolution

The specifications of the thermometer are first compared with the clinical factors required for a clinical thermometry system.

The measurements were carried out with a plastic container (PVC) filled with either water or ultrasonic gel. One part of the container was covered with a thin foil. In this way, the

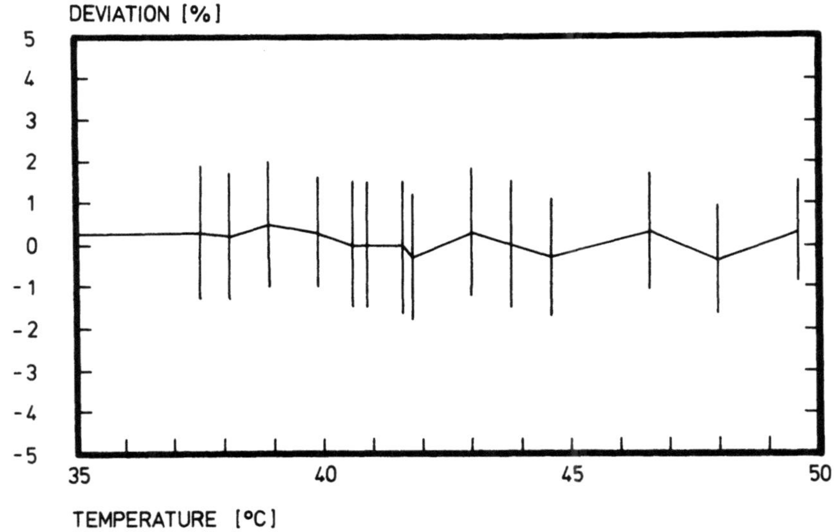

Fig. 5. Linearity test of the microwave thermometry unit between 35 °C and 55 °C. The results are standardized to thermistor measurement; the average deviation is shown by the *error bars*

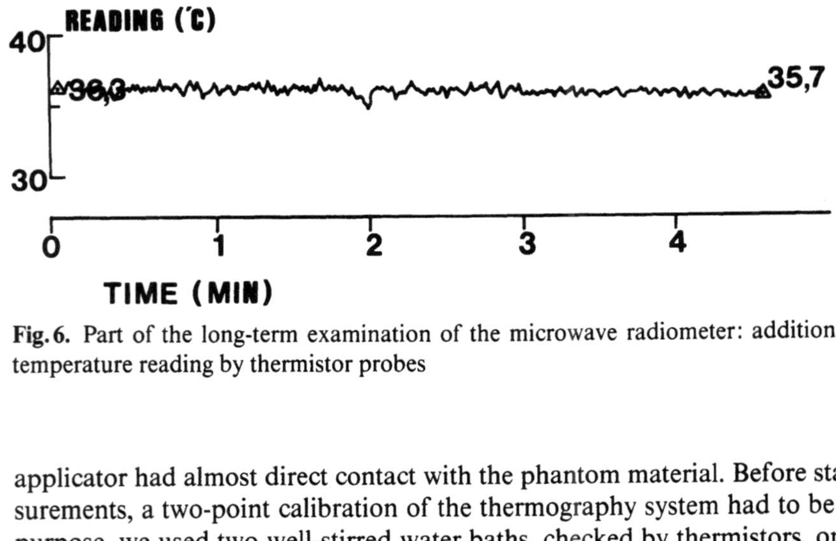

Fig. 6. Part of the long-term examination of the microwave radiometer: additional checks of the temperature reading by thermistor probes

applicator had almost direct contact with the phantom material. Before starting the measurements, a two-point calibration of the thermography system had to be done. For this purpose, we used two well-stirred water baths, checked by thermistors, one at 20 °C and the other at 60 °C.

The first experiment was the examination of the linearity of the displayed temperature in water that ranged from 35 °C to 50 °C. The measured temperature was compared with a thermistor (Fenwal Electronics Inc, Farmingham, Mass., United States) probe measurement (Fig. 5). The graph in Fig. 5 shows the results of the linearity test, standardized to the thermistor measurement. The error bars show the average deviation of the display. The next plot, illustrates a part of the long-term examination (Fig. 6). The plotter was directly connected to the microwave receiver and a graph of a time-dependent temperature profile was drawn. The temperature of the water bath was about 36 °C. The temperature of the water was checked by a thermistor probe every 5 min. The maximum deviation was 1 °C, the average deviation 0.5 °C. The average of the integral of the displayed temperatures with a sequence of 1 s indicated a deviation of 0.1 °C over a period of 10 s. It is evident that the result of the measurement can be improved by using a microprocessor.

Spatial Resolution

The spatial resolution cannot be checked with one fixed antenna but with a moving antenna or with a combination of several antennae using the overlapping profile. Furthermore, the application of several frequencies is necessary to obtain information of the temperature distribution, depending on the various depths. The lateral resolution of this system is approximately 1.5 cm.

Response Time

The measuring period is adjusted to 12 s. Theoretically, approximately 1.2 s is needed to obtain a resolution of one-tenth of a degree according to the formula (Lüdeke 1983):

$$M = \frac{k^2(T_0 + T_R)^2}{B\sigma^2} \tag{2}$$

where M is measuring time, K is system constant for a Dicke-type radiometer ($K \sim 2$), T_0 is temperature of the object, T_R is temperature of the receiver, B is bandwidth (400 MHz), and σ is temperature resolution (0.1 °C).

The much longer period of 12 s is caused by the switch on and off of the receiver and generator. The error of this measurement, that is, the cooling down during this period, amounts to 0.2 °C tested on a static phantom.

Influence of Inhomogeneities

With regard to in vivo application of microwave thermography in a hyperthermia system, we performed some checks on the influence of inhomogeneities on the result of the measurement.

In a homogeneously heated water bath, we examined the effect of fat slices on the temperature measurement. The 5- to 20-mm-thick slices were moved away from the antenna in 1-cm steps (Fig. 7). Figure 7 shows the error that is dependent on the distance between the antenna and fat slice. For a 20-mm slice in direct contact with the applicator, we found an error of more than 60 °C. The reason for this error is the high reflectivity and the low emissivity of fat.

The situation at the antenna-phantom interface explains the error of the measurement. The temperature of a homogeneously heated phantom is T_0. The microwave radiation emitted toward the surface is partly reflected at the interface. One part of this radiation, determined by the emissivity (E) of the phantom material, reaches the antenna. There is a similar situation in the antenna: the receiver temperature flow is partly reflected at the interface and partly emitted into the phantom. The resulting temperature (T) seen by the receiver is (Fig. 8):

$$T = T_0 E + T_R R \tag{3}$$

where E = emissivity and R = reflectivity.

Due to the conservation of energy the reflection of the power and the absorbed power add up to 100%:

$$T_R = T_R R + T_R A$$
$$1 = R + A \tag{4}$$

together with the reciprocity of all parts of the object

$$E = A$$
$$1 = E + R \tag{5}$$

where A = absorption.

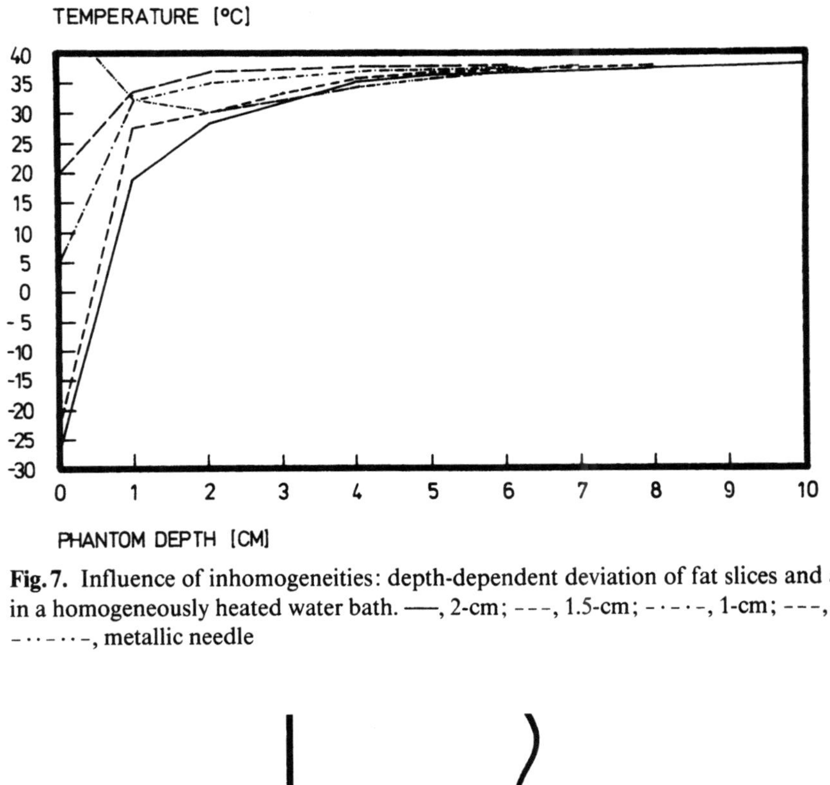

Fig. 7. Influence of inhomogeneities: depth-dependent deviation of fat slices and a metallic needle in a homogeneously heated water bath. —, 2-cm; - - -, 1.5-cm; - · - · -, 1-cm; - - -, 0.5-cm fat slices; - · · - · · -, metallic needle

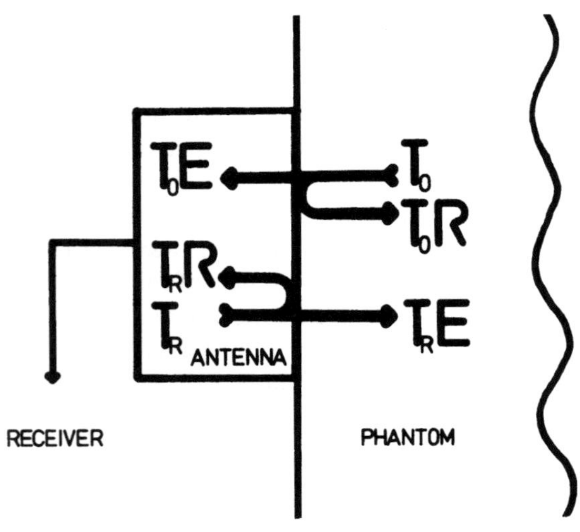

Fig. 8. Schematic diagram of the interface between the antenna and the phantom

Equation (3) is equal to

$$T - T_0 = R(T_R - T_0) \tag{6}$$

It can be seen that there is no measurement error if $T_R = T_0$, i.e., the temperature T seen by the receiver equals T_0, the temperature of the object. Our radiometer is adapted to muscle tissue, i.e., T_R does not follow T_0; thus the different reflectivity of different tissues is going to influence the error.

During investigations carried out at the Philips Laboratory the problem was solved by simultaneous measurement of the apparent temperature and the reflectivity of the object, to allow calculation of its actual temperature. At Leroy in Lille the so-called zero method was developed: in this the receiver temperature T_R follows the object temperature T_0. The error disappears when T_0 equals T_R.

The upper line in Fig. 7 represents the influence of a hollow needle in which a probe may be used as an additional measurement device. Deviations of more than 5 °C are possible. When using microwave thermography, even the metallic leads of the probes will produce errors. If additional measurements are required, systems working with fibers are necessary.

Experiments with Nonhomogeneously Heated Volumes

Further experiments were aimed at examining the power regulation dependent on the temperature. The phantom used was a container filled with ultrasonic gel to simulate the tissue. The microwave generator was started at the lowest power of 5 W. The chosen temperature was 43 °C, the heating and measurement sequence 1 min and 12 s (Fig. 9). As shown in Fig. 9, the generator was regulated up to 80 W in steps of 0.5 dB. After having reached a temperature of 38 °C, the power was reduced gradually. The reduction of the power was much too slow and thus the chosen temperature was exceeded by 3 °C. This effect is also displayed in Fig. 10a, b, which shows the time-dependent temperature in a

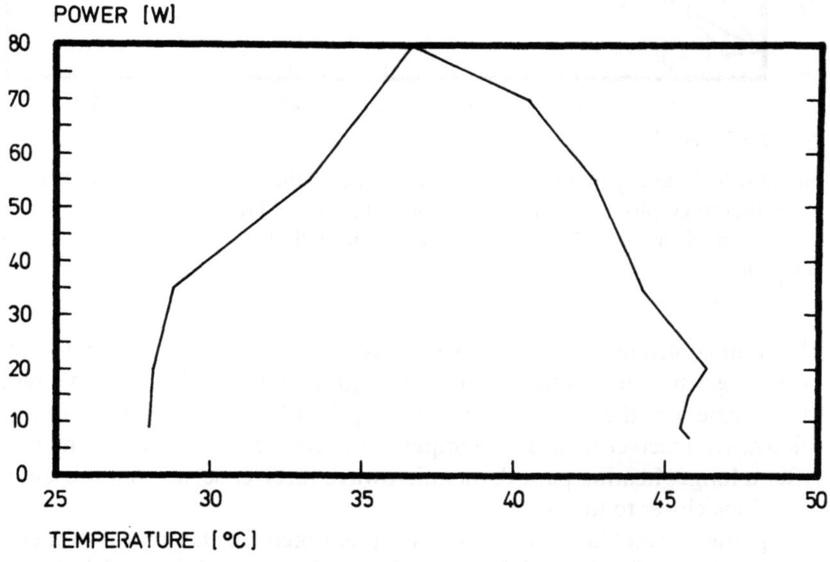

Fig. 9. Temperature-dependent power regulation of the microwave generator

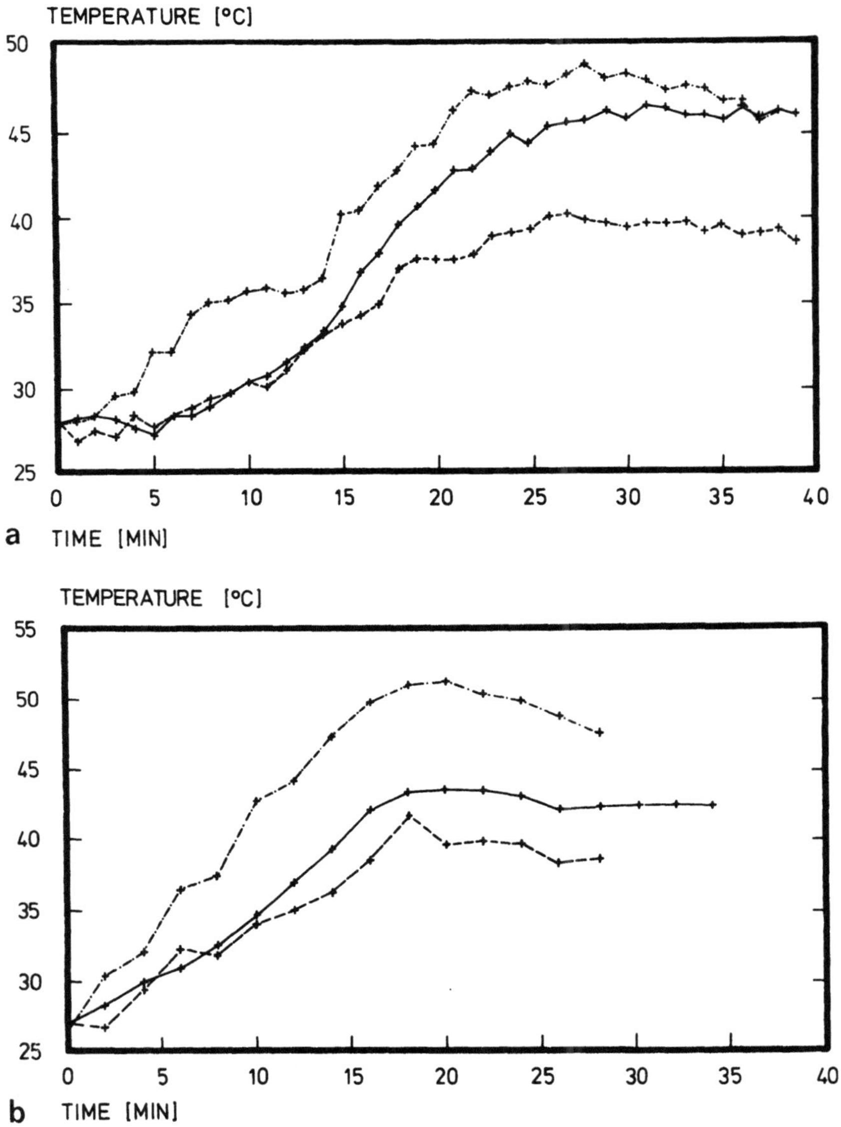

Fig. 10 a, b Time-dependent temperature profile of the hyperthermia system controlled by microwave thermography (——). **a** Further measurements with thermistor probes at a depth of 2 cm (-·-·-) and 4 cm (---). **b** Further measurements with thermistor probes at a depth of 1 cm (-·-·-) and 3 cm (---)

phantom controlled by the microwave receiver and checked by two thermistor probes. In both diagrams, there is no relation between the displayed microwave receiver result and measurement of thermistor probes at a depth of 1-4 cm. During the first few minutes, the microwave-receiver-measured temperature represents the conditions in deeper regions. After a longer heating period, the microwave receiver seems to represent the temperature in regions closer to the surface.

A plane parallel layer model has been adopted for theoretical modeling (Bardati and Solimini 1983). The flux of the thermal radiation toward the surface is determined by the contribution of each layer. For a model with constant temperature T_i per layer, the surface temperature is:

$$T = \sum_i E_i T_i \quad (7)$$

i.e., in a nonhomogeneous temperature distribution the thermal radiation detected by the antenna is an integral of all the volume elements of different temperatures and emissivities. The emission of the thermal radiation toward the surface is determined by the reduction of the intensity caused by the absorption. For a plane wave without reflecting interfaces, the decrease follows an exponential function. In general, for a nonhomogeneous model (temperature and material), a weighting function has to be introduced. This function has to consider the depth-dependent influences produced by the reflection at the interfaces of the layers.

In our experiment, the absorption of the microwave radiation coming from deeper regions causes a stronger reduction of the signals than the more intensive signals coming from the hotter regions close to the surface. This effect explains the higher weighting of the surface signals. One possible solution is the application of several additional frequency ranges, for example, in order to obtain depth-dependent correcting factors, i.e., to obtain information about the unknown temperatures T_i.

Conclusions

The conclusions of our preliminary examination of a microwave thermography system working on the frequency band of 100-500 MHz are summarized. The depth dependency of the measured temperature must be improved using scan methods, i.e., the application of several frequencies in order to evaluate weighting factors. A better spatial resolution of the temperature is only attainable when several applicators are used. Furthermore, the problem of the dependency of the displayed temperature on different tissues must be solved. Microwave thermography can only be applied if measurements can be carried out even though the emissivities of the tissues are not precisely known or may vary from one treatment session to the other.

References

Andersen JB, Baum A, Harmark K, Heniel L, Rasmark P, Overgard J (1984) A hyperthermia system using a new type of inductive applicator. IEEE Trans Biomed Eng 31 (1): 21-27

Bardati F, Solimini D (1983) Radiometric sensing of biological layered media. Radio Sci 18 (6): 1393-1401

Bliek L, Heizmann M (1976) Erwärmungsfehler und Zeitverhalten von Thermistor-Temperaturaufnehmern für medizinische Elektrothermometer. PTB Mitt 86: 399-405

Christensen DA (1983) Thermometry and thermography. In: Storm FK (ed) Hyperthermia in cancer therapy. Hall, Boston, p 223

Dewey WC, Hopwood LE, Sapareto SA, Gerweck LG (1977) Cellular responses to combinations of hyperthermia and radiation. Radiology 123: 463

Divrik AM, Roemer RB, Cetas TC (1984) Interference of complete tissue temperature fields from a few measured temperatures. An unconstrained optimization method. IEEE Trans Biomed Eng 31 (1): 150-160

Edrich J (1984) Methods and results of breast cancer detection using correlated infrared and multi-depth microwave thermography. Internationaler Thermographiekongreß, Luzern
Gerthsen C, Kneser HO (1969) Physik, 10th edn. Springer, Berlin Heidelberg New York
Hand JW (1984) Thermometry in hyperthermia. In: Overgaard J (ed) Hyperthermic oncology, vol 2. Taylor and Francis, London, pp 299-308
Lüdeke KM (1983) Grundlagen der medizinischen Mikrowellenthermographie. In: Engel JM, Flesch U, Stüttgen G (eds) Thermologische Meßmethodik. Notamed, Baden-Baden, pp 140-161
Myers PC, Sadowsky NL, Barrett AH (1979) Microwave thermography: principles, methods and clinical applications. J Microwave Power 14: 105-115
NCRP (1981) Radiofrequency electromagnetic fields. National Council of Radiation Protection and Measurement, Washington, report no 67
Nguyen DD, Chivé M, Leroy Y, Constant E (1980) Combination of local heating and radiometry by microwaves. IEEE Trans Instrum Meas 29 (2)
Nilsson P (1984) Physics and technique of microwave-induced hyperthermia in the treatment of malignant tumors. Nilsson Per, Lund
Plancot M (1983) Contribution à l'étude théorique, expérimentale et clinique de l'hyperthermie microonde contrôlée par radiométrie microonde. Thesis, Université des Sciences et Techniques, Lille
Plancot M, Chivé M, Giaux G, Prevost B (1984) Thermal dosimetry in microwave hyperthermia process based on radiometric temperature measurements: principles and feasibility. In: Overgaard J (ed) Hyperthermic oncology, vol 1. Taylor and Francis, London, pp 863-866
Porter RA, Miller HH (1978) Microwave radiometric detection of breast cancer. (Conference Record Boston Mass) IEE, New York
Vaguine VA, Christensen DA, Lindley JH, Walston TE (1984) Multiple sensor optical thermometry system for application in clinical hyperthermia. IEEE Trans Biomed Eng 31 (1): 168-172

Microwave Radiometry for Temperature Monitoring in Biological Structures: An Outline

F. Bardati and D. Solimini

Diparimento di Ingegneria Elettronica, Università di Roma "Tor Vergate,"
Via Orazio Raimondo, 00173 Rome, Italy

The determination of temperatures in the human body both provides valuable support in diagnostics and is a necessity during hyperthermic treatment. In the diagnostic application, since the temperature of neoplastic tissues is higher than that of the surrounding normal tissues of the host, it is important to be able to detect a localized increase in temperature. In hyperthermic applications the temperature in the tissues must be continuously monitored to ensure that the required heating rate in the tumor bulk is attained without concurrent damaging effects on the surrounding normal cells. This contribution is concerned mainly with the interpretation of data in passive microwave sensing of nonhomogeneous biological structures, by summarizing relevant aspects both of a model of the radiative transfer in the living tissues and of the inversion technique through which the temperature information can be extracted from the radiometric data (Bardati and Solimini 1983).

Model of Emission

Two different approaches can be followed to investigate microwave emission from nonhomogeneous media (Schmugge and Choudhury 1981). In the "incoherent" approach, the intensity of the emitted radiation is obtained by solving the radiative transfer equation, while the "coherent" approach makes use of solutions of Maxwell's equation with the pertinent boundary conditions. Thermal emission is intrinsically an incoherent process. However, reflections which may be caused by nonrandom inhomogeneities in a stratified emitting medium produce interference effects, so that the emerging radiation exhibits partial coherence. Choice of either model relies on the characteristic thickness of the inhomogeneities (Carver 1977). Since typical thicknesses are in the millimeter or, at most, in the centimeter range, the effect of multiple reflections from the boundaries of the different kinds of tissues can be important. For this reason, a coherent approach must be followed to evaluate microwave emission from the assumed model.

In the following, for the sake of simplicity we shall model the subcutaneous region of tissues as a half-space $z<0$, where both the temperature and the physical properties vary only with distance z from the body surface. By Fourier analyzing (Bekefi 1966) the electromagnetic emission of radiation from the thermal body in the loss-less half-space $z>0$, the spectrum of the brightness temperature $T_{Bp}(\omega, \mathbf{k})$ is obtained, where ω is the angular frequency of a monochromatic radiometric channel which measures the time-averaged elec-

Recent Results in Cancer Research. Vol 101

tromagnetic flux (proportional to T_{Bp}), having polarization p and propagating at angle $\cos \vartheta = \hat{\mathbf{z}}\hat{\mathbf{k}}$ ($\mathbf{k} = \hat{\mathbf{k}}\ \omega/c$; c is the speed of light in the half-space $z > 0$).

According to the Rayleigh-Jeans approximation, the contribution to T_{Bp} of a layer of tissue at depth z and of thickness Δz is $T(z) \cdot \Delta\tau_p(\omega, \mathbf{k}, z)$, where $T(z)$ is the physical temperature and $\Delta\tau_p$ is a proportionality factor. By adding partial contributions from all depths z, the following equation is obtained in the limit $\Delta z \to 0$:

$$T_{Bp}(\omega, \mathbf{k}) = \int_0^{\varepsilon_p} T(z)\, d\tau_p(\omega, \mathbf{k}, z) \tag{1}$$

where ε_p is the body emissivity. When the natural structures, as in the biological case, can be described by arrangements of several electrically homogeneous layers separated by planes across which the dielectric constant is discontinuous, expressions for τ_p and ε_p can be readily obtained, as has been shown by Bardati and Solimini (1984a).

The brightness temperature of the biological structure can be alternatively written as:

$$T_{Bp}(\omega, \mathbf{k}) = \int_{-L}^{0} T(z)\, W_p(\omega, \mathbf{k}, z)\, dz \tag{2}$$

where $W_p = d\tau_p/dz$ and the lower limit of integration, $-L$, indicates the depth within the tissues beyond which the contribution to the brightness becomes negligible, i.e., $\tau_p(z < -L) \approx 0$. Note that $W_p(\omega, \mathbf{k}, z)$ is the brightness temperature which is measured when the temperature is null everywhere but for a very thin hot spot of value T at depth z.

As an example, consider an emitting half-space at a uniform temperature T. From Eq. (1) $T_{Bp} = \varepsilon_p T$, as is expected. ε_p depends on the thickness and on the dielectric permittivity and conductivity of layers, as well as on frequency, polarization, and angle of observation. When the body temperature is not uniform (this is the case in living tissues), full Eq. (2) must be used in order to predict the thermal emission from the body. Knowledge of the weighting function for the observed structure is necessary. Figure 1 illustrates a typical example of weighting functions for a skin-fat-muscle arrangement and for three values of frequency and 1-GHz bandwidth of the radiometric channel.

It is interesting to note from Fig. 1 that, generally, the same measured brightness may correspond to different temperature distributions in the tissues. For instance, a 1.5-GHz radiometer does not distinguish between two localized hot spots of the same value at 3 or 30 mm. The above example shows that one measurement is not sufficient for temperature reconstruction, even in a monodimensional approximation of tissues and of temperature profiles. It is apparent, therefore, that microwave thermography requires several independent measurements for adequate use in clinical applications.

Temperature Reconstruction

It has been suggested that the spatial distribution of the temperature can be determined quantitatively from a convenient set of measurements, provided suitable algorithms are available to extract the searched for data from the measurements. This inverse problem is defined by Eq. (2), where the physical temperature $T(z)$ is the unknown in the Fredholm integral equation of the first kind (2) and a finite discrete set of measurements is given. This set can be generated by measuring the brightness temperature of the biological structure at various frequencies, polarizations, and angles of observations. Moreover, noise in

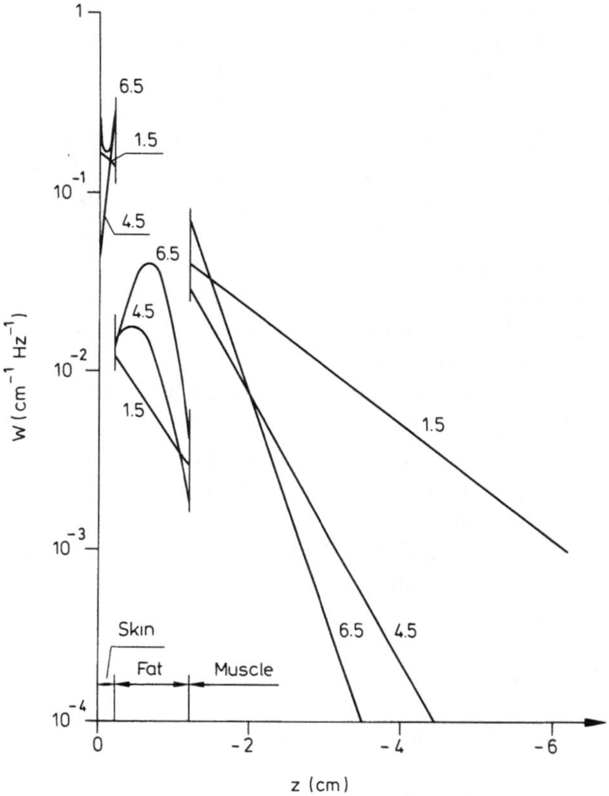

Fig. 1. Weighting function W versus depth z for a skin-fat-muscle arrangement and for the indicated values of frequency and 1 GHz of bandwidth of the radiometric channel. Direction of observation perpendicular to the tissue layers

the radiometric data must be taken into account. It should be observed that this problem is ill conditioned and the solution is affected by intrinsic numerical instability. Moreover, since noise in radiometric data is present, suitable inversion techniques must be used to circumvent such difficulties. The following is computational scheme that has been recently proposed.

First the integral Eq. (2) is reduced in matrix form, by means of /■/ expansion of the searched for temperature on a suitable M-dimensional basis of functions, $b_i(z)$, $i=1, \ldots, M$ (Bardati et al. 1983):

$$T(z) = \mathbf{b}^{\tau}(z) \cdot \boldsymbol{\vartheta} \tag{3}$$

where $\mathbf{b}^{\tau}$ is the transpose of vector $\mathbf{b}$, having components $b_i(z)$; and $\boldsymbol{\vartheta}$ is the vector of expansion coefficients. Performing integrations in Eq. (2) yields the matrix equation $\mathbf{T}_B = \mathbf{W}\boldsymbol{\vartheta}$, where $\mathbf{T}_B$ is the N-dimensional vector of measurements and $\mathbf{W}$ is a $N \times M$ matrix. In order to take noise in the radiometric data into account, a vector $\boldsymbol{\nu}$ must be added to measurement vector $\mathbf{T}_B$:

$$\mathbf{W}\boldsymbol{\vartheta} = \mathbf{T}_B + \boldsymbol{\nu} \tag{4}$$

Equation (4) must now be solved with respect to $\boldsymbol{\vartheta}$ by using a suitable inversion technique, which prevents the noise $\boldsymbol{\nu}$ from substantially corrupting the sought for solution.

Of the several inversion methods that have been proposed for the solution of Eq. (4), the Kalman filtering estimation algorithm has proven to be a fairly effective technique in terms of both accuracy of retrievals and attainable spatial resolution (Basili et al. 1981). In addition, since it is a recursive technique, Kalman filtering is well suited for use in monitoring the temporal evolution of temperature profiles, as is required in the relevant case of hyperthermic treatments of tumor tissues.

In this procedure, the choice of the basis used for expansion (3) is of great importance. Indeed, such a basis should be able to represent the temperature distributions using only few terms in (3), even when localized hot spots have to be considered. Orthogonal polynomials (e.g., Laguerre polynomials) and prolate functions have been used. More recently (Bardati and Solimini 1984b), the basis of singular functions of the integral Eq. (2) has been proposed. As is known, this basis well represents that part of the temperature distribution which contributes more effectively to the measured brightness.

Special care should also be taken when planning the measurements. A convenient procedure for generating the required set of independent data is to measure the brightness temperature of the biological structure at a given set of different frequencies. The number N of frequencies should be kept small, not only to reduce the complexity and cost of the system and the acquisition and computation time, but also to reduce the effects of ill-conditioning that tend to increase with increasing dimensions of the matrix **W**. On the other hand, the choice of the frequencies is crucial, since the interdependence of measurements must be minimized to reduce the unstabilizing effect of ill-conditioning, or, to maximize the information content of the assigned number of measurements.

References

Bardati F, Solimini D (1983) Radiometric sensing of biological layered media. Radio Sci 18: 1393-1401

Bardati F, Solimini D (1984a) On the emissivity of layered materials. IEEE Trans Geosci Remote Sensing 22: 374-376

Bardati F, Solimini D (1984b) Modelling emission from biological tissues: application to microwave thermography. Open Symposium on Interaction of Electromagnetic Fields with Biological Systems, XXI URSI General Assembly, Florence, August 28-September 5

Bardati F, Conventi U, Solimini D (1983) Determination of temperature profiles in biological media by microwave radiometry. Proc Int URSI Symp, Santiago de Compostela, August 23-26, pp 681-683

Basili P, Ciotti P, Solimini D (1981) Inversion of ground-base radiometric data by Kalman filtering. Radio Sci 16: 83-91

Bekefi G (1966) Radiation processes in plasmas. Wiley, New York

Carver KR (1977) Radiometric recognition of coherence. Radio Sci 12: 371-379

Schmugge TJ, Choudhury BJ (1981) A comparison of radiative transfer models for predicting the microwave emission from soils. Radio Sci 16: 927-938

Fiber Fabry-Perot Thermometer for Medical Applications

R. Kist, S. Drope, and H. Wölfelschneider

Fraunhofer Institut für Physikalische Messtechnik, Heidenhofstrasse 8,
7800 Freiburg i. Brsg., FRG

Introduction

One of the specific properties of fiber optic sensors is their capacity to perform in electromagnetically contaminated environments. In the biomedical field of hyperthermia, i.e., the controlled heating of biological tissues by microwave irradiation, there is a need for continuous and high-resolution temperature measurement in the microwave field (Hahn 1982). The temperature sensor signal should be suited for controlling the microwave generator itself in order to follow a well-defined temperature versus time curve of the tissue under treatment.

Conventional temperature sensors made from metallic or semiconductor materials have the disadvantage that the sensor element and the necessary wires heat up in the microwave field and distort the electromagnetic power distribution. This may cause wrong measurements as well as an inhomogeneous temperature distribution, which can lead to so-called hot spots within the tissue.

In the present paper, a temperature sensor is described which has specific characteristics to serve the needs of hyperthermia systems:

1. No microwave field deformation and no self heating
2. Short and thin sensor element, which is suited for local and invasive measurements
3. Measuring range of about 35°–55 °C with a resolution of better than 0.1 °C

Description of the Sensor

The concept of the Fiber Fabry-Perot (FFP) interferometer (Yoshino et al. 1982; Kist and Sohler 1983) has been adopted for the temperature sensor element. The ends of a short piece (11.6 mm in the present case) of monomode fiber were polished and dielectrically coated to provide an optical FFP resonator with a finesse F of about 10 and a free spectral range of 1.8×10^{-2} nm. As shown in the sensor system schematics (Fig. 1), this FFP is attached to a single-mode fiber (SMF), which transports light from the laser diode (LD) (AlGaAs, Hitachi HL7801E, $\lambda = 790$ nm) to the FFP and guides the light reflected by the FFP via a 3-dB all-fiber directional coupler to the detector (D). The laser light is collimated, passed through an optical isolator, and focused to the input fiber of the coupler.

The reflected signal I_R is schematically shown in the insert of Fig. 1 as a function of the temperature-dependent optical length $n(T) \cdot L(T)$, with $n(T)$ being the refractive index of

Recent Results in Cancer Research. Vol 101

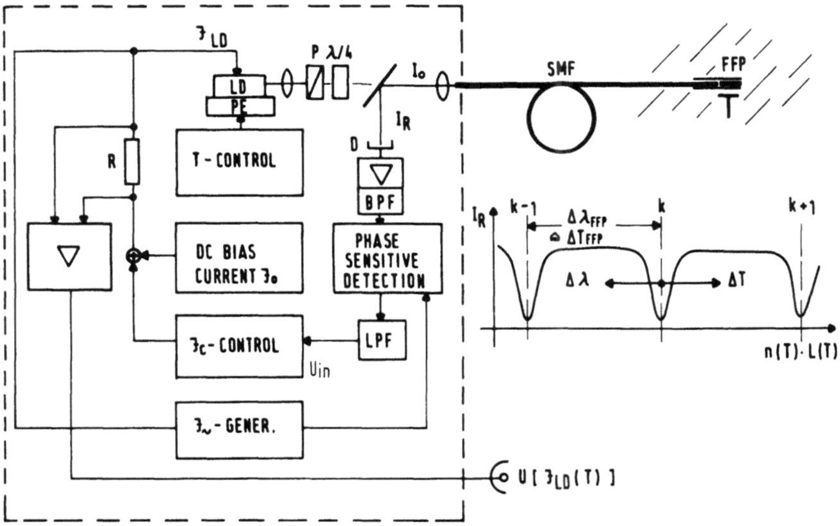

Fig. 1. Schematics of the FFP temperature sensor

the FFP core and $L(T)$ the FFP length (11.6 mm). The sequence of the reflection minima of order $k-1$ to $k+1$, for example, can be produced either by changing $n(T) \cdot L(T)$ via a temperature change ΔT or by scanning the wavelength λ of the laser via the injection current. The latter method is used in the example of the oscillogram (Fig. 2), which displays the transparency maxima (lower trace) and the reflection minima (upper trace) of the FFP. In terms of injection current, the neighboring peaks are spaced by $\Delta J_{LD}=2.8$ mA. The corresponding temperature and wavelength intervals are $\Delta T=3.2$ °C and $\Delta\lambda=1.8\times10^{-2}$ nm, respectively.

The basic idea of the temperature sensor is to compensate the effect of a temperature change ΔT which would shift the FFP output toward the neighboring order, say from k to $k+1$, by a suitable wavelength change $\Delta\lambda$, so that the signal I_R is locked to the reflection minimum of order k. Thus the net change

$$\delta\Phi=\delta\Phi_n\cdot L+\delta\Phi_\lambda=\frac{4\,\pi}{\lambda}\,\delta(n\cdot L)-\frac{4\,\pi n L}{\lambda^2}\,\delta\lambda \tag{1}$$

of the round trip phase $\Phi=4\,\pi\, nL/\lambda$ of the FFP light wave is controlled to zero. The metrological task then consists of

1. Stabilizing the laser wavelength via stabilization of the laser temperature to within a few 10^{-5} nm or a few millikelvins, respectively,
2. Locking to a particular order of the FFP signal, for example, the one that corresponds to normal body temperature,
3. Controlling the laser wavelength with the FFP sensor element as the spectral reference.

Temperature stabilization to within a few millikelvins has been achieved with a modified version of an existing control electronics system (Schumann and Tietgen 1984), which provides a stabilized current to the Peltier cooler, to which the laser diode is attached.

The wavelength control makes use of a stabilization scheme with phase-sensitive detection for controlling the laser injection current. In this method, the laser diode current I_{LD}

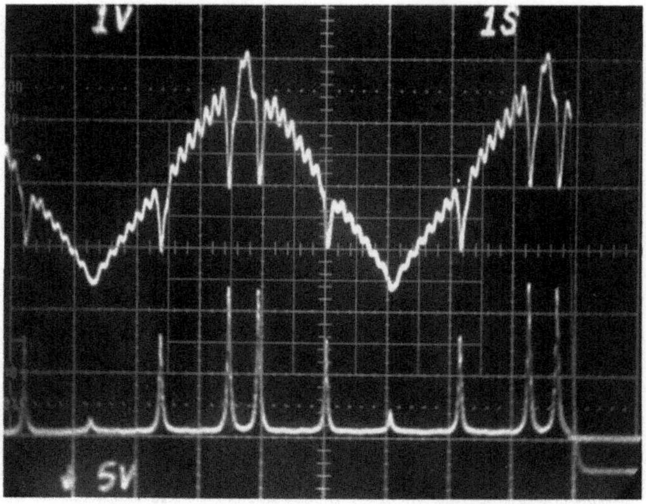

Fig. 2. Oscillogram with FFP transparency maxima *(lower trace)* and reflection minima *(upper trace)*

is composed of a bias current I_0, a controlled DC current I_c, and an AC component $I\sim$. The latter oscillates at 5 kHz and slightly modulates the wavelength of the laser radiation. This wavelength modulation is transformed by the FFP reference element into an intensity modulation, which is detected by the photodetector D and amplified (A 1). The modulation component contained in the reflection signal I_R is isolated by a band pass filter (BPF) and phase sensitively detected with respect to the phase of the modulation signal $I\sim$. There is a zero transition of the phase difference between the detected 5-kHz component and the $I\sim$ signal if the modulation drifts from one side to the other of the reflection peak, i.e., from negative to positive slope of the optical signal. Correspondingly the voltage U_{in} provided by the integrating low-pass filter (LPF) goes through zero if the phase difference passes through zero. U_{in} is fed to the J_c-control unit, which controls the DC laser current component and hence the laser wavelength - with the laser-active layer temperature as the intermediate parameter - such that U_{in} is tuned to zero. The current sum $I_0 + I_c$ is measured across a precision resistor R with a precision amplifier (A 2) to provide the voltage $U[J_{LD}(T)]$, which is a measure of the laser wavelength and is calibrated against the temperature T to be measured.

This method has been successfully used to stabilize the frequency of an AlGaAs laser to within a few 100 kHz (corresponding to 2×10^{-5} nm) with respect to an FFP that served as spectral reference element (Wölfelschneider and Kist 1984). Since the laser current and hence wavelength control rely on locking to the reflection minimum, the method does not depend on intensity variations, i.e., possible bending loss in the lead fiber, coupling losses, etc.

Results

The FFP sensor was inserted into a water bath 20 mm in diameter and 30 mm in depth together with two Pt 100 temperature transducers, whose relative accuracy is ± 1 mK. The water bath temperature was varied by a set of three Peltier elements, typically between 25° and 45 °C. Figure 3 shows the calibration curve of the FFP sensor. The current interval ΔI_{LD}, as derived from the voltage $U[J_{LD}(T)]$ (see Fig. 1), is plotted against the FFP temper-

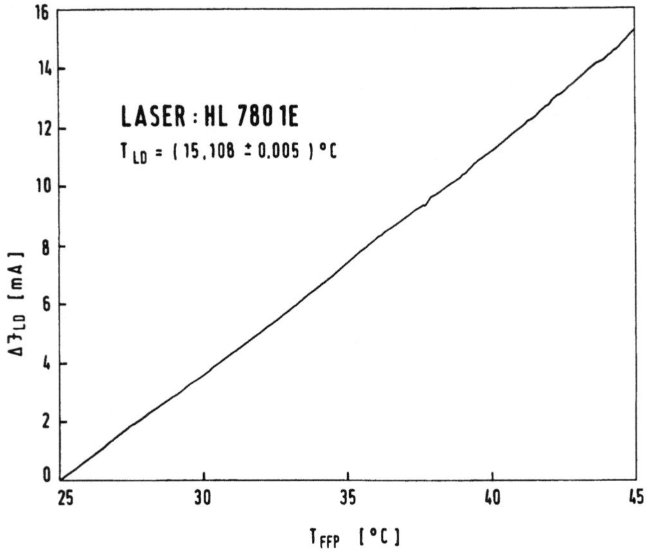

Fig. 3. Injection current change ΔJ_{LD} against temperature T_{FFP} calibrated by means of a Pt 100 transducer

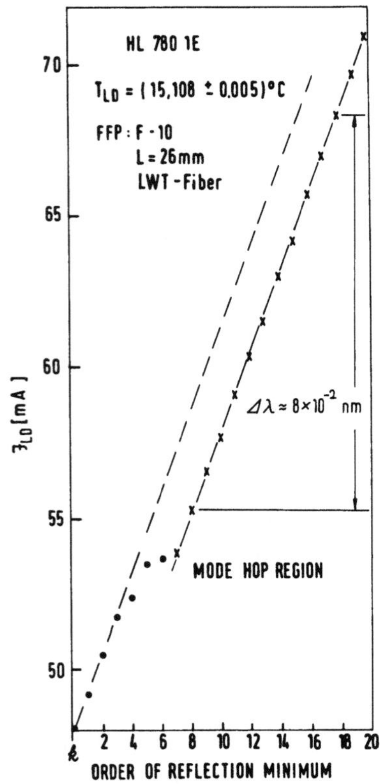

Fig. 4. Injection current J_{LD} for consecutive reflection minima

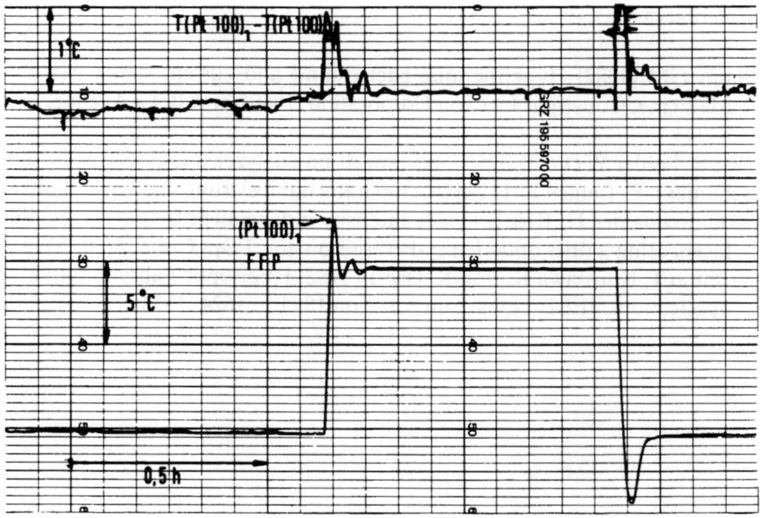

Fig. 5. Comparison of FFP temperature values with Pt 100 temperature over a period of 2 h

ature T_{FFP}, as measured by the calibrating Pt 100. The curve shows that the FFP temperature sensor covers the range of 20 °C, which has been specified for the envisaged hyperthermia application.

Starting at a given FFP order, say k, at $I_{LD} = 48$ mA, the current values for consecutive reflection minima have been plotted as shown in Fig. 4. There is a mode hop region around 53 mA, but the interval from 55 to 71 mA is straight and linear, thus allowing for undisturbed FFP sensor operation in this interval.

The resolution of the system is actually limited by the temperature stability, which is of the order of ± 5 mK over the injection current range 55–71 mA. This corresponds to a resolution of about 5×10^{-2}K, whereas the accuracy of the laser wavelength control tuned to the FFP reflection minimum corresponds to a resolution of the order of 1 mK.

Figure 5 displays in the upper trace the temperature difference $T(\text{Pt } 100)_1 - T(\text{Pt } 100)_2$ of the two Pt 100 probes, which are arranged together with the FFP probe in the water bath in a triangular geometry with a few millimeters spacing.

The lower traces of Fig. 5 compare the calibrated FFP thermometer with one of the Pt 100 probes over a period of 2 h. The temperature of the water bath is switched between the two stabilized temperature values 34.7 °C and 44.6 °C. Switching is accompanied by a temperature overshoot and slight oscillation, which provides a total temperature interval of almost 17 °C.

The curves demonstrate that the FFP temperature signal follows the $(\text{Pt } 100)_1$ temperature to within 0.1 °C, except for situations where the temperature distribution in the water bath is not homogeneous, especially after bath temperature switching.

After the successful demonstration of this FFP temperature sensor, future work will focus mainly on a suitable coating of the sensor tip (with outer diameter of 0.5 mm or less) and integration into a microwave hyperthermia system.

Acknowledgment. The authors would like to thank W. Stein and F. Horn for building the laser temperature control unit and W. Ott for helpful discussion as well as technical assistance. This work has been supported by the Bundesministerium für Forschung und Technologie, Bonn.

References

Hahn GM (1982) Hyperthermia, background and current status. Stanford University School of Medicine, Copyright Luxtron Corporation, 1060 Terra Bella Avenue, Mountain View, California 94043

Kist R, Sohler W (1983) Fiber-optic spectrum analyzer. J Lightwave Technol 1: 105-110

Schumann F, Tietgen KH (1984) Temperaturstabilisierung von Laserdioden. Elektronik 11: 59-62

Wölfelschneider H, Kist R (1984) Intensity-independent frequency stabilization of semiconductor lasers using a fiber optic Fabry-Perot resonator. J Opt Commun 5: 53-55

Yoshino T, Kurosawa K, Itoh K, Ose T (1982) Fiber-optic Fabry-Perot interferometer and its sensor applications. IEEE J Quantum Electron 18 (10): 1624-1633

Temperature Measurements by Nuclear Magnetic Resonance and Its Possible Use as a Means of In Vivo Noninvasive Temperature Measurement and for Hyperthermia Treatment Assessment

B. Knüttel and H. P. Juretschke

Bruker Medizintechnik, Silberstreifen, 7512 Rheinstetten/Karlsruhe, FRG

Introduction

It is well known that the control of hyperthermia treatment for deep-seated tumors is exceptionally difficult. At present, the increase in temperature produced by irradiation is monitored by the introduction of temperature sensors at specific points in the body. With this technique, the stress the patient inevitably has to endure is considerable. Furthermore, the possibility of the introduction of the temperature sensors causing a metastasis cannot be excluded. Temperature is the first parameter which suggests itself as a means to monitor hyperthermia treatment. Therefore it would seem worthwhile to look for alternative, noninvasive temperature measurement methods. Additionally, metabolic parameters which change upon irradiation may be suitable indicators of the success of hyperthermia treatment. It is, for example, known that hyperthermia treatment influences metabolic parameters as well as blood flow and pH values. Those effects which may occur during hyperthermia achieved by irradiation are: (1) temperature increase, (2) changes in metabolite concentrations, (3) changes in metabolic process rates, and (4) production of radicals. All the quantities listed here are, theoretically at least measurable by nuclear magnetic resonance (NMR). In order to indicate the potential of this technique, some of the more commonly occurring terms used in NMR will now be explained.

Introduction to NMR

Although for the past 25 years NMR has been an indispensable analytical tool for chemists and biochemists, it has become known to a wider range of scientists only in the past 4-5 years. This expansion has been largely due to new fields of application in medicine, above all NMR tomography and in vivo spectroscopy. While the former technique is very suitable for the production of images, competing to a certain extent with computer tomography, in the latter technique an attempt is made to apply the spectroscopic techniques of chemistry and biochemistry to in vivo studies of human metabolism.

As excellent NMR textbooks are available (James 1975; Gadian 1982), we will limit ourselves to a brief enumeration of some NMR parameters it is convenient to use for temperature measurements. In an NMR spectrum, the chemical shift value δ of a resonance yields information on the electronic and magnetic environment of the corresponding nucleus at the atomic level, the area of the resonance being related to the number of nuclei present.

Recent Results in Cancer Research. Vol 101

Upon absorption of energy by any spin system (resonance condition), this energy is dissipated into the surrounding lattice with a characteristic time constant, termed the spin-lattice relaxation time T_1. Additionally, during the irradiation process a magnetization transverse to the magnetic field H_0 is built up. The decay of this magnetization, a purely entropy-driven process, is governed by the spin-spin relaxation time T_2.

Both quantities, T_1 and T_2, depend in a very complex manner on the chemical structure of the molecule and on dynamic processes in and around the observed molecule, both intracellular and extracellular. Thus it is possible to examine, along with chemical exchange processes, also diffusion and flow phenomena in biological systems.

These four parameters, i. e., chemical shift, signal intensity, and T_1 and T_2, may be influenced by other factors, such as the presence of radicals, the water concentration, or the temperature:

Control of Hyperthermia Experiments by NMR Methods

Parameter	*Influenced by*
T_1, T_2	radical, H_2O, T
δ	pH, T
Signal intensity	Metabolite,
Magnetization transfer	$\frac{\delta\,(\text{Metabolite})}{\delta t}$, T

These factors in turn may be influenced by hyperthermia treatment. Hence, these four NMR parameters could be suitable monitors for assessing the effect of an irradiation experiment.

In Fig. 1, the effect of irradiation on metabolite concentrations as seen by ^{31}P NMR is exemplified for a subcutaneously implanted Dunn osteosarcoma tumor before and after

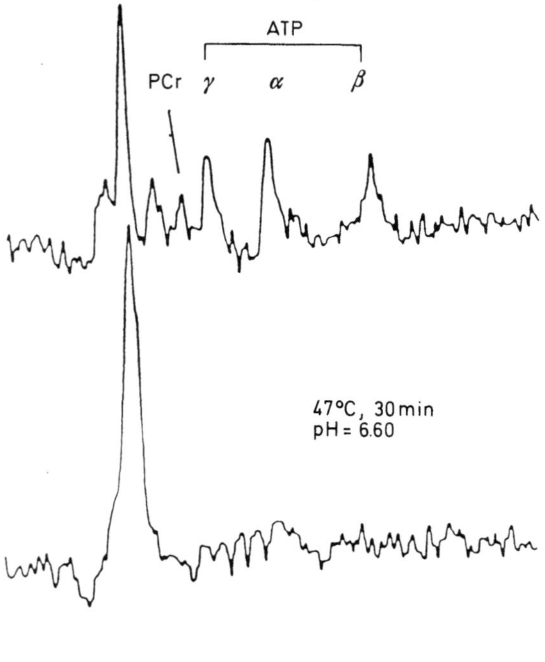

Fig. 1. ^{31}Phosphorus NMR spectra (512 scans) of two subcutaneously implanted Dunn osteosarcoma tumors (monitored before and after hyperthermia treatment at 47 °C for 30 min). (Ng et al. 1982)

hyperthermia treatment (taken from Ng et al. 1982). In the spectrum measured upon irradiation no ATP signals are to be seen while the inorganic phosphate signal increases in area. These changes in metabolite concentration indicate an extensive tumor cell kill and, hence, may be suitable parameters to check the effect of a hyperthermia treatment.

Temperature Measurement Parameters

In analytical high-resolution NMR various temperature measurement methods are currently in use. Most are based on the determination of chemical shift changes upon variation of temperature as shown in Fig. 2, where two 300-MHz spectra of ethylene glycol at temperatures of 300 K and 350 K are displayed. A shift of the OH-line by 100 Hz (2 Hz/ °C) with respect to the methyl signal is observed. This method of temperature determination is widely used in chemistry since it is a direct method and the resonance frequency can be determined very accurately.

In Table 1 the most commonly used thermometric compounds and their corresponding fields of application are listed. The third column shows the dependence of the chemical shift on temperature. We have restricted ourselves here to those compounds used in the positive temperature range. The next column shows the sensitivity of the chemical shift to temperature variation. The frequency variation per degree Celsius was calculated for a

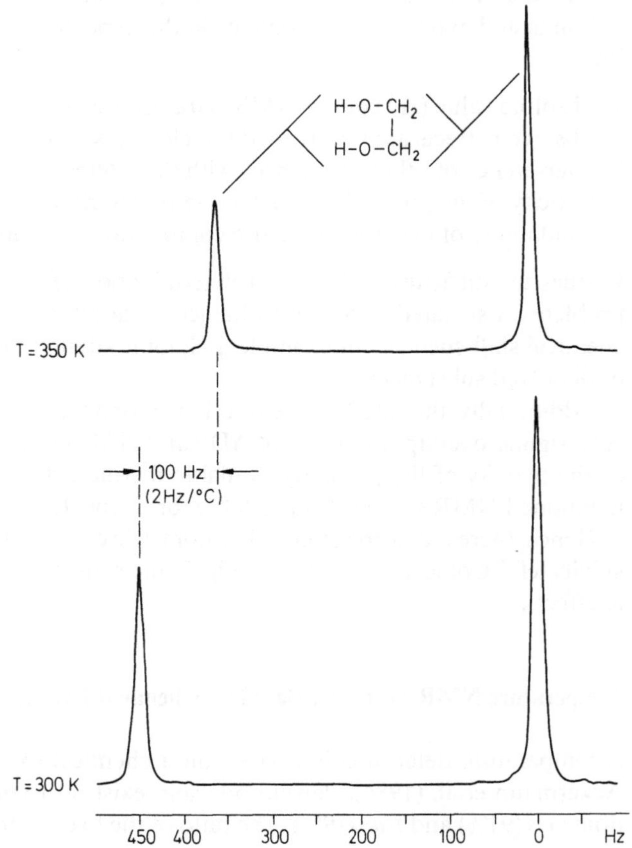

Fig. 2. Temperature dependence of chemical shift in ethylene glycol. Ethyleneglycol in DMSO-d_6 at 7 T Field (≙ 300 MHz ^{1}H)

Table 1. Data for some NMR standards used for temperature measurements (chemical shift)

Nucleus	Thermometric compound	Temperature dependence of the chemical shift $\Delta\delta$ (ppm)	Sensitivity of δ (Hz/ °C)[a]	Temperature parameter
^{1}H	Methanol	$T=468.1-181.0\,\Delta\delta$	~ 0.6	$OH \leftrightarrow CH_3$
^{1}H	Ethyleneglycol	$T=466.0-169.4\,\Delta\delta$	~ 0.6	$OH \leftrightarrow CH_2$
^{13}C	Iodomethane	$1/T=0.01611-0.00057\,\Delta\delta$	~ 1	$CH_3I \leftrightarrow TMS$
^{31}P	Mg ATP	$T=-2.5732\,\Delta\delta+726.7$	~ 0.5	$\alpha P \leftrightarrow \beta P$
^{59}Co	Co (acac)$_3$ in $CDCl_3$	$T=0.0134\,\Delta\delta$	~75	^{59}Co (X°C) $\leftrightarrow$ ^{59}Co (0 °C)

[a] Referred to $B_0=2.3488$ T (≙ 100 MHz ^{1}H resonance)

field strength of 2.4 T. The last column indicates the temperature-dependent parameter used, usually the difference in chemical shift between two specific lines.

Included are the methanol and ethylene glycol probes (Günther 1973) as well as the alkyl halides and ^{59}Co compounds used in ^{13}C NMR work (Vidrine and Peterson 1976; Levy et al. 1980).

The major drawback to the temperature determination through chemical shift changes in the required accuracy of the frequency measurement, about 1 Hz or less for the usual nuclei (cf. Table 1). In in vivo NMR measurements relatively broad resonances are usually observed and this requirement is therefore difficult to meet.

Limits and experimental problems in this type of temperature measurement are as follows:

1. Absolute value ($\Delta\delta$) of the NMR parameter change
2. Observed effects are intertwined too closely with factors other than temperature
3. Interference of other resonances with the interesting ones (ATP↔ADP, NAD)
4. Toxicity of the presently available thermometric substances
5. Availability of new thermometric compounds with large chemical shift changes

Besides the difficulty in the exact determination of $\Delta\delta$ mentioned above, there are also problems associated with the influence of additional parameters which also alter the chemical shift such as, for example, pH, ionic strength of the medium, and concentration of dissolved substances.

Additionally, the interference of other resonances with the interesting ones [e.g., some ATP signals overlap with those of ADP and NAD in ^{31}P spectra (Gupta and Gupta 1980)], or the toxicity of the presently available thermometric substances, render several of the mentioned NMR standards unsuitable for in vivo temperature determination.

Hence, there is a need for new thermometric compounds with a strong temperature sensitivity [cf. $^{59}Co(acac)_3$ in $CDCl_3$ in Fig. 5] and satisfactory water solubility but without toxic effects.

Temperature NMR Standard Based on Chemical Exchange

A temperature determination based on a chemical exchange process was suggested by Ackermann et al. (1984). Perfluorodecalin exists at room temperature in two conformations: *cis* (91%) and *trans* (9%). The ratio of the two conformations shows a linear temperature dependence whose temperature sensitivity is greater than that of the previously mentioned thermometric compounds.

Fluorocarbons, administered as neat liquids or as constituents of artificial blood, are ideal thermometric fluids. They exist in vivo as inert, discrete microphases; their spectra are largely unaffected by their microchemical environment. The temperature effect is easily discernible. Their intrinsic NMR sensitivity is excellent. Oxygen partial pressure, while it has a definite effect on T_1, does not affect temperature measurement.

Temperature Measurement Through Water Resonance

Both the chemical shift δ and the spin lattice relaxation time T_1 of the water protons are temperature dependent.

The changes in the chemical shift of the water resonance upon variation of temperature are due to changes in the water structure, i.e., strength of hydrogen bonding, lifetime of these bonds, etc.

In an organism, water molecules in different environments contribute to the water resonance, thus increasing its linewidth. Because of the different environments, different temperature coefficients for the different water "subspecies" must also be expected. Thus a specific water subspecies has to be selected in order to have a thermometric substance with a defined temperature dependence. By taking advantage of the different T_2 relaxation times of water protons in the various environments, such a selection is possible. Using the CPMG (Carr-Purcell-Meiboom-Gill) pulse train, the water molecules with a long T_2-time may be selected, rendering a narrow line, the resonance position of which can be determined accurately.

In this context the temperature dependence of the T_2 time of water should be mentioned. For pure, degassed water, a change in T_2 of 75 ms/°C in the range 30°-50 °C was determined.

The next problem to be tackled is the need for a reference or standard signal in the spectrum to which the changes in resonance position may be referred. The resonance of fat protons seems to be a suitable choice. It is easily detectable and far less sensitive to temperature than water resonance. Hence, the difference in chemical shift between the fat and the selected water proton signals could be a suitable parameter for in vivo temperature measurements. Especially attractive is the inherent noninvasive and nontoxic character of this method.

The use of the spin-lattice relaxation time T_1 as a temperature indicator is hampered by the high sensitivity of this parameter to paramagnetic substances (like O_2) or other radicals. This is especially true, since due to the uneven distribution of O_2 in the body a varying influence has to be expected.

Ways of Measuring the Various Parameters

All of the previously mentioned quantities, such as chemical shift, relaxation times, spin density, and chemical exchange, can be measured by means of NMR. An instrument equipped to measure these physical phenomena usually consists of the following components:

Magnet System

This central unit serves to magnetize the nuclear spins. The size of the field is determined by the sort of nuclei to be examined, the size of the sample, and the available financial resources.

Radiofrequency or Spectrometer Electronics

These components produce the exciting radiofrequency field and then detect the weak NMR signal with high sensitivity.

Computer System

This unit takes care of the production of the corresponding complex pulse program, processes the NMR signal, and carries out the image processing to improve the signal-to-noise ratio or improve the image quality.

An example of such a system is shown in Fig. 3. The spectrometer, including the computer unit, and the separate magnet unit are easily recognized as the type of system that is required for in vivo spectroscopy. In this case, a magnet of 2.4 T and 40-cm bore is shown as being ideal for in vivo examination of experimental animals. Correspondingly larger magnets are also available for the whole body range without alteration of the electronic unit.

A system such as that shown here offers NMR imaging as well as the possibility of in vivo spectroscopy. The former technique is in the present case of especial interest since it offers the possibility of localizing a tumor without disturbing or influencing any irradia-

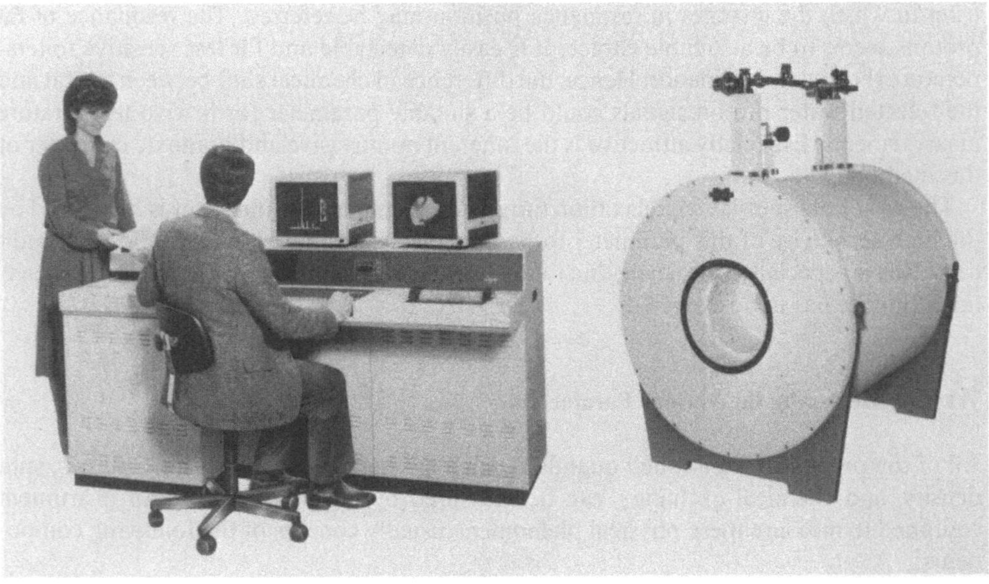

Fig. 3. NMR computer and magnet system

tion experiment which may have to be carried out. Damadian was the first to demonstrate that cancerous and healthy cells can be distinguished on the basis of their different relaxation times. Besides other factors, the basis of the higher water content of the cancerous cells can explain this effect.

This effect can be demonstrated on a sagittal head scan of a midline tumor. This tumor is pathoanatomically a pilocystic astrocytoma. In Fig. 4a-d the same tumor (white sphere in the middle) is represented by the transformation of various echoes (1st, 9th, 17th, and 25th), and hence various delay times, of a CPMG sequence. With corresponding T_2 discrimination, it is possible in the ideal case to differentiate between necrotic tissue, tumor, and lesions. A danger-free method for long-term monitoring (screening) is thus available, providing a means of control during the irradiation process. In particular, a multidimensional relaxation time measurement can be carried out with this low-resolution system without the need to change the operating conditions.

In addition, with such a system - after alteration of the operating conditions - in vivo spectroscopic examinations can be carried out. For this, one selects with the help of newly developed techniques a defined area of tissue in order to obtain the corresponding quantities such as chemical shift or amplitude variation in the resolved spectrum (i.e., the position of interest is measured by high-resolution NMR). NMR is therefore a very promising technique which in various ways permits localization of the measurement and with which it is possible to conduct long-term monitoring of the irradiation process by simultaneous or time-deferred measurement of the desired screening parameter.

Summary

In the foregoing we have tried to give a broad survey of the parameters which are of importance for irradiation experiments and which can be measured by NMR. Since it is the temperature change during irradiation that is of immediate interest, we have tried to emphasize the ways in which this quantity can be measured. This has shown that temperature measurement by means of the chemical shift has experimental limits as well as the fact that overlapping signals may cause problems. Hence, more experiments must be carried out in order to clarify the possibilities of its use. Although experimentally this is no easy task, it is feasible. In particular, the possibility of determining the temperature by external markers introduced into the tissue should be studied. The development of new nontoxic thermometric compounds with greater sensitivity would be a great step forward.

The possibility of determining the temperature through the relaxation times of water represents a real alternative, especially since this can be carried out by low-resolution NMR. Additional experiments are necessary in order to see whether the sensitivity attainable is satisfactory.

Chemical exchange processes and changes in metabolite concentration could also be used to measure the temperature or the effect of an irradiation experiment.

In conclusion, one can say that the measurement of control parameters (especially for irradiation experiments by means of NMR) represents a difficult experimental problem. It does not promise success in all cases but probably represents the only noninvasive measurement possibility. For this reason, wide-ranging experiments should be initiated in order to obtain definitive results.

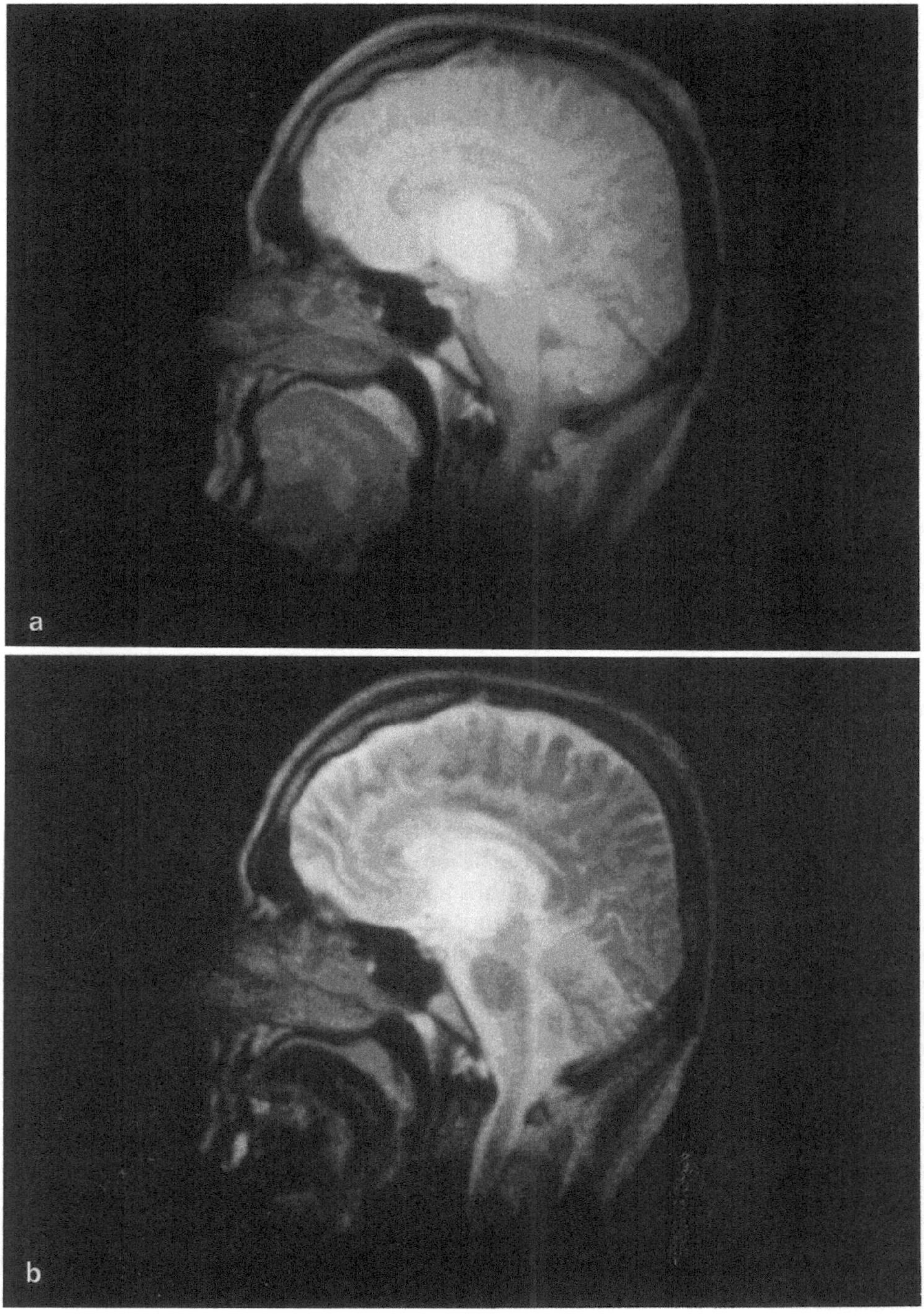

Fig. 4a–d. Sagittal head-scan of a midline tumor with NMR imaging

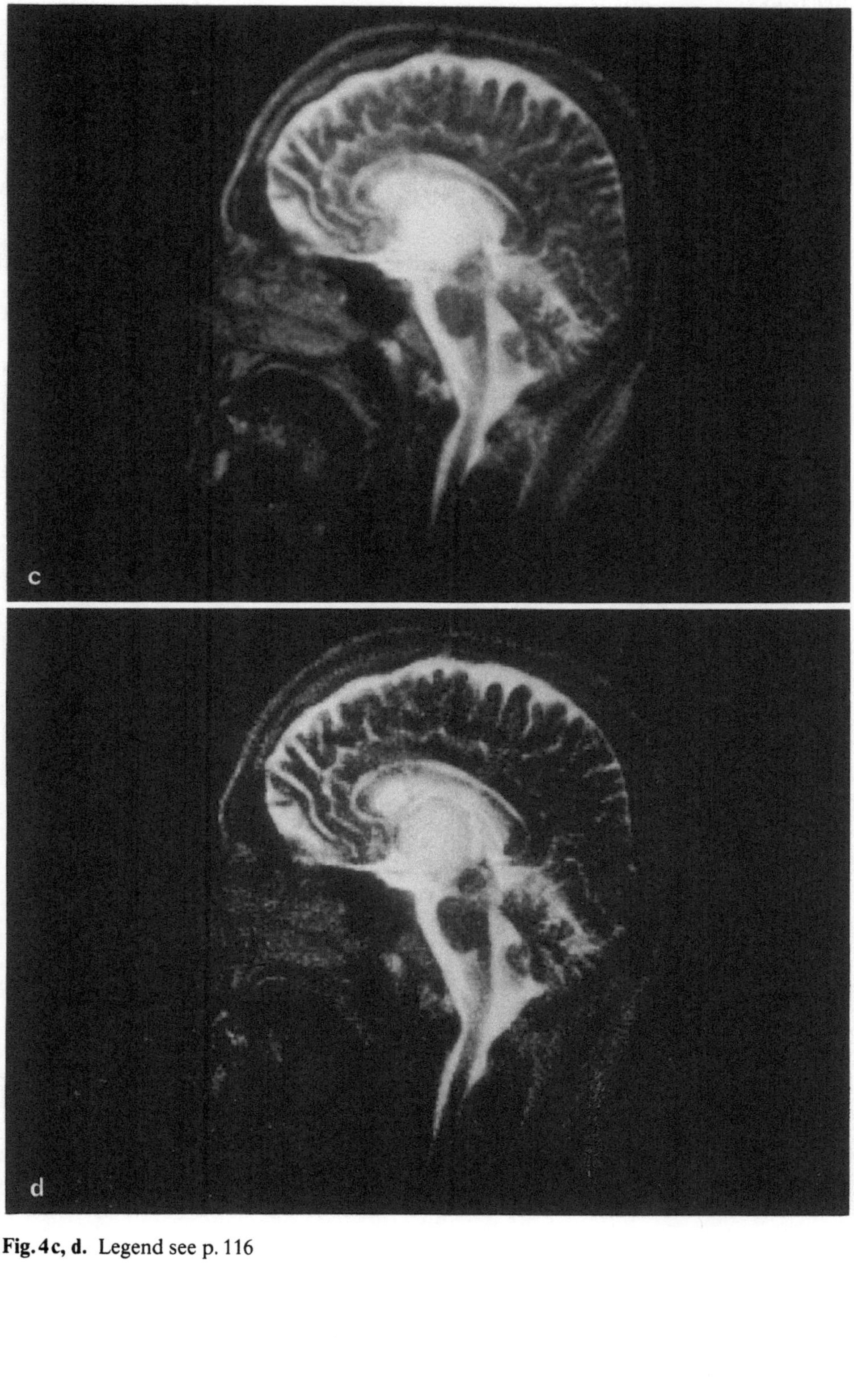

Fig. 4 c, d. Legend see p. 116

References

Ackermann JL, Clark LC, Thomas SR, Pratt RG, Kinsey RA, Becattin F (1984) NMR thermal imaging. Proceedings of the 3rd Annual Meeting of the Society of Magnetic Resonance in Medicine, New York, pp 1-2

Gadian DG (1982) NMR and its applications to living systems. Oxford University Press, Oxford

Günther H (1973) NMR Spektroskopie. Thieme, Stuttgart

Gupta RK, Gupta P (1980) A magnesium (II) ATP thermometer for ^{31}P NMR studies of biological systems. J Magn Reson 40: 587-589

James TL (1975) NMR in biochemistry: principles and applications. Academic, New York

Levy GC, Bailey JT, Wright DA (1980) A sensitive NMR thermometer for multinuclei FTNMR. J Magn Reson 37: 353-356

Ng TC, Evanochko WT, Hiramoto RN, Ghanta VK, Lilly MB, Lawsan AJ, Corbett TH, Durant JR, Glickson JD (1982) ^{31}P NMR spectroscopy of in vivo tumors. J Magn Reson 49: 271-286

Vidrine DW, Peterson PE (1976) Simultaneous temperature measurement during acquisition of pulsed Fourier transformed carbon-13 magnetic resonance spectra. Anal Chem 48: 1301-1303

Hyperthermia Treatment Planning

J. J. W. Lagendijk and J. Mooibroek

Academisch Ziekenhuis Utrecht, Instituut voor Radiotherpie van de Rujksuniversiteit,
Catharijnesingel 101, 3511 CG Utrecht, The Netherlands

Introduction

The planning of hyperthermia treatment, i.e., the prediction of absorbed power distribution and resulting temperature distribution in a given tissue volume, is a prerequisite for the successful clinical introduction of hyperthermia as a standard curative treatment of malignant tumors. For the selection of adequate treatment techniques and treatment protocols and for the proper evaluation of treatment results, it is necessary to have information about the actual small-scale temperature distribution in tissue. The real time calculation of the temperature distribution during actual treatment, while utilizing measured temperature data to optimize the temperature fit, can be of great use in controlling the feedback of the treatment process.

The first step in hyperthermia treatment planning is the calculation of the real three-dimensional absorbed power distribution in tissue produced by the heating methods applied. These calculations are hindered by the capacity of most present-day computer systems and by the lack of available data on the three-dimensional anatomical structures of each individual patient. However, it is expected that within several years modern 16- and 32-bit, large-memory, personal "mainframe" computers will help to solve the computing problems.

Anatomical data, especially of the important soft-tissue structures, are being made available through NMR imaging (Bakker and Vriend 1984). Two-dimensional approximations of absorbed power distribution in structured tissues heated with radiofrequency and microwave techniques have been made (van den Berg et al. 1983; Iskander et al. 1982). Care must be taken in applying the results obtained with these models on real three-dimensional patient geometries (Lagendijk and de Leeuw, this volume, p. 18). **E**-fields perpendicular to fat (bone)-muscle (organ) interfaces can produce severe overheating of the fat (bone) structures. These overheating problems are eliminated by the parallel **E**-field orientation related to the tissue interfaces in the two-dimensional computational models.

The second step in hyperthermia treatment planning is the calculation of the resulting temperature distribution. In normal vascularized tissues, the temperature distribution is dominated by heat transport due to blood flow (Jain et al. 1979; Chen and Holmes 1980; Lagendijk 1982; Lagendijk et al. 1984). This greatly complicates the development of computational models. Generally, the time-dependent temperature distribution in vascularized tissues is described by the conventional "bioheat transfer" equation (Pennes 1948).

Recent Results in Cancer Research. Vol 101

Thermal models based on a numerical solution of the "bioheat transfer" equation have been developed by Strang and Patterson (1980), Bowman (1981), Hynynen et al. (1981), Hand et al. (1982), Ozimek and Cetas (1982), Strohbehn (1982), Lagendijk et al. (1984), and others.

As will be demonstrated in the following, it is fundamentally incorrect to apply this conventional theory to the small-scale heat transfer problems in hyperthermia (Lagendijk 1984).

To evaluate the difficulties in describing the enormous influence of blood flow on tissue heat transport, we shall divide the vessel network into three phases according to vessel size ranging from large main arteries and veins to small capillaries. The description of each phase is specific in tissue heat transfer theory.

An analytical evaluation of the heat transfer process in vascularized structured tissues is made impossible by the great complexity of the problem.

We shall try to evaluate the heat transfer problems related to each of the three phases using a finite difference numerical computer model in order to arrive at the basis of a new numerical theory to describe the actual temperature distribution in real patient anatomies.

The major problem of how to obtain sufficient blood flow data from each individual patient will direct the development of the new numerical theory.

The clinical consequences of the influence of blood flow heat transport on the actual temperature distribution in hyperthermia practise will be discussed.

Theory Phantoms or "Tissues" Without Blood Flow

In phantoms and in tissues without blood flow, temperature distribution can be calculated by solving the following differential equation plus associated boundary and possible initial conditions:

$$\rho C_p \frac{\delta T}{\delta t} = \mathrm{div}\,(K \,\mathrm{grad}\; T) + P + M \tag{1}$$

with ρ, C_p, and K the density, the specific heat, and the thermal conductivity of the tissue, respectively. T is the temperature. The two production terms P and M describe the rate of heat production per unit volume due to heating and metabolic heat production, respectively.

This equation can easily be solved numerically using finite difference heat balance techniques (Croft and Lilley 1977). With this method, the tissue is divided into small, mostly rectangular elements (Fig. 1). The temperature of each element is described by its center (node) temperature. Assuming that the temperature of all the elements has been known at a given time t, the temperature of the elements can be calculated at time $t+\Delta t$ by considering the heat flow between the elements related to the known temperature at time t and the heat production in the elements in time interval Δt. The total heat flow toward element (0) is given by:

$$\psi_f = \sum_{i=1}^{6} \frac{K(i)+K(0)}{2} \frac{A(i)}{L(i)} \,(T(i) - T(0)) \tag{2}$$

with $A(i)$ being the surface between element (0) and element (i) and $L(i)$ the distance between node (0) and node (i). The interface between different tissues must be located exactly between two elements. In element (0) there is heat production:

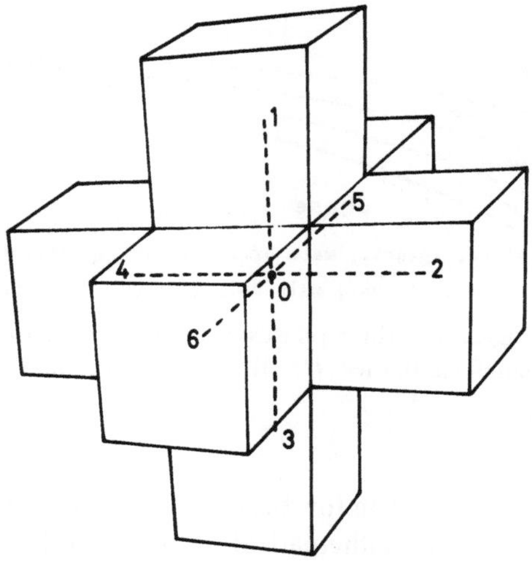

Fig. 1. Cubical element structure of the finite difference thermal model

$$\psi_p = V(0)\,(P(0) + M(0)) \tag{3}$$

with $V(0)$ being the volume of element (0). The total heat $\psi_f + \psi_p$ entering element (0) results in a temperature change in this element described by:

$$\varphi_t = \Delta t\,(\psi_f + \psi_p) = V(0)\,\rho C_p\,(T(0)' - T(0)) \tag{4}$$

with $T(0)'$ being the new temperature of element (0) at time $t+\Delta t$.

In this way, it is possible to calculate the temperature of all the elements at time $t+\Delta t$ from the old temperatures at time t. By repeating this procedure, the temperature distribution can be followed in time, starting with an initial (arbitrary) temperature distribution (for instance, 37 °C for all elements) at time $t=0$.

With this technique, which is called the explicit forward heat balance technique, the partial differential Eq. (1) is solved. Because of the physical transparency of this method, it is, as shall be shown, fairly easy to introduce discrete blood vessels in the computational model. A detailed description of the use of this method is given in Lagendijk et al. (1984).

Theory Description: Blood Flow

Generally, the temperature distribution in vascularized tissues is described by the "bioheat transfer" equation (Pennes 1948). In this theory, the influence of blood flow is described by the addition of a heat sink term B to Eq. (1):

$$\rho C_p \frac{\delta T}{\delta t} = \mathrm{div}\,(K\,\mathrm{grad}\,T) + P + M - B \tag{5}$$

B is the amount of heat withdrawn (heat sink) from each tissue volume by the blood flow represented by:

$$B = V_{bl}\,Cp_{bl}\,(T - T_{ar}) \tag{6}$$

where V_{bl} is the perfusion rate and T_{ar} is the temperature of the main supplying artery. The basic assumption of this theory is that the blood enters the local tissue volume at arterial temperature and leaves this volume at the local tissue temperature.

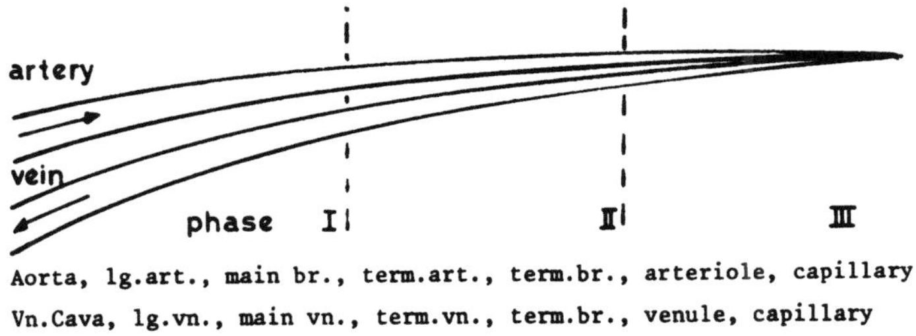

Fig. 2. The three phases of blood flow according to vessel size, from main arteries and veins *(I)* to small capillaries *(III)*. Branches are omitted for clarity

The reason for this equation remaining the basis of most thermal modeling for 36 years lies in its mathematical simplicity and in its intelligent mathematical form. It fails in its description of heat transfer processes in vascularized tissues. The combination of heat production terms (P and M) and a heat sink term (B), which are all spatially variable, together with the fact that the solid tissue heat transfer contribution by conduction is relatively unimportant, makes possible the fit of almost every measured tissue temperature distribution. The values of B found with this fitting process are of no prospective value and thus useless for hyperthermia treatment planning systems.

The main objection against the conventional "bioheat transfer" theory is that it neglects the following aspects: (1) the heat transport related to the mass transport of blood, (2) the actual temperature of blood entering the local tissue volume, (3) the individual (cooling) influence of large vessels, and (4), last but certainly not least, the fundamental importance of the entire venous vessel network.

To understand the real influence of blood flow on tissue heat transfer, we first have to consider the structure of the tissue vessel network. We shall divide the vessel network into three phases (Fig. 2) according to actual physiological length in relation to thermal equilibrium length of the individual vessels. Thermal equilibrium length is defined as the length over which the temperature difference between the blood in the vessel and the surrounding tissue is reduced by a factor e, for the situation that a vessel enters a tissue region heated to a uniform temperature. Phase I now consists of large vessels, both arteries and veins, with thermal equilibrium length much longer than their actual physiological length. Phase II consists of vessels with thermal equilibrium length of the order of actual vessel length and Phase III consists of small vessels whose equilibrium length is small in comparison with vessel length.

A detailed evaluation of the heat transfer processes related to each vessel-type phase requires a computational model that describes the influence of discrete vessels and discrete vessel networks on tissue heat transfer.

Theory: Discrete Vessels

To evaluate the influence of discrete vessels on heat transport, we incorporate these vessels in the numerical finite difference model (FDM).

A vessel with radius r is divided into elements with length L, equal to the node distance in the FDM (Fig. 3). We define a mixing cup temperature $< T_{bl} >$, which represents the temperature that would result if the blood of an element were thoroughly mixed to a uni-

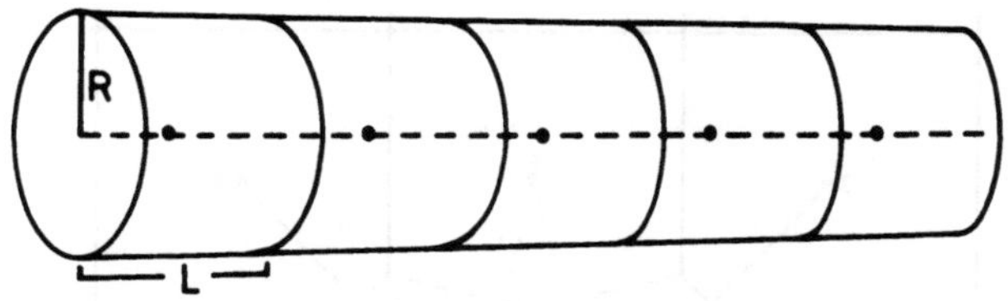

Fig. 3. Vessel with radius R divided into elements with length L equal to the node distance of the FDM. The blood in each element has a mean temperature $< T_b(i) >$

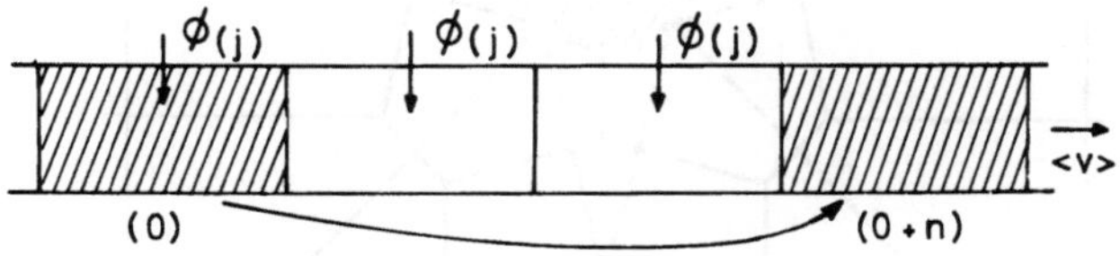

Fig. 4. Heat and blood flow in time interval Δt in a vessel of radius r and flow velocity $< v > = nL/\Delta t$

form temperature. The heat flow through the vessel wall with a known temperature $T_w(0)$ of the blood vessel element (0) in question is given by:

$$\psi_{bl} = h_{bl} A_{bl} (T_w(0) - < T_{bl}(0) >) \tag{7}$$

where A_{bl} is the vessel wall surface of the element ($A_{bl} = 2\,\pi r L$) and h_{bl} the heat transfer coefficient which describes the heat flux through the vessel wall. The heat transfer coefficient h_{bl} is given for a laminar flow vessel by Drew et al. (1936a, b) and Lagendijk (1982):

$$h_{bl} = 3.66\ K_{bl}/2\,r \tag{8}$$

where K_{bl} is the thermal conductivity of the blood.

In forming the heat balance for a vessel we must realize that, besides the heat transfer from the tissue through the vessel wall, there is a heat flow in the vessel related to the mass flow of the blood. We derive the heat balance for blood element (0) (Fig. 4). At time t, the temperatures of all blood elements are presumed to be known. In time interval Δt, blood element (0) has moved to blood vessel element $(0+n)$, with $n = < v > \Delta t/L$. Along this path the blood has exchanged heat with the surrounding tissue boundary elements, which have known vessel wall temperature. The total heat flow toward the moving blood element in time interval Δt is given by:

$$\varphi_t = \sum_{j=0}^{0+n-1} \psi_{bl}(j) \Delta t/n = \Delta t/n \sum_{j=0}^{0+n-1} A_{bl}(j) h_{bl} (T_w(j) - < T_{bl}(0) >) \tag{9}$$

This heat results in a temperature change of the blood element in question described by:

$$\varphi_t = V_{bl}(i)\, \rho_{bl}\, Cp_{bl} (< T'_{bl}(0+n) > - < T_{bl}(0) >) \tag{10}$$

where $< T'\ (0+n) >$ is the new blood temperature at time $t + \Delta t$ of blood vessel element $(0+n)$. Cp_{bl} and ρ_{bl}, respectively, are the specific heat and the density of the blood and V_{bl} is the volume of blood element (0). This describes the temperature change of the blood as well as the heat transport related to the mass flow of the blood. The three-dimensional rectangular FDM must be modified in such a way that the blood vessel can be incorporat-

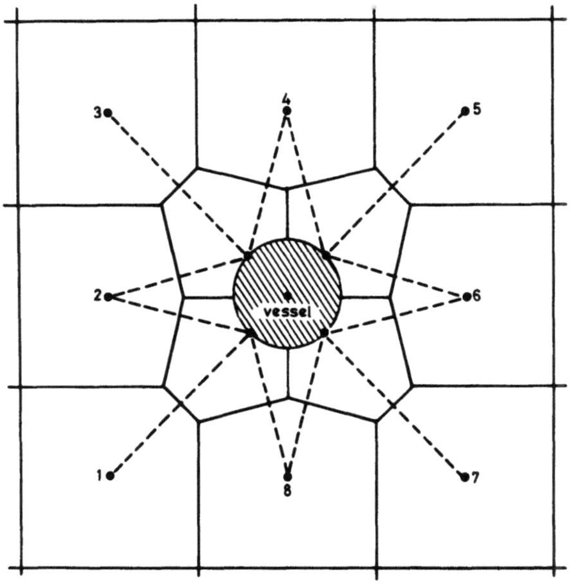

Fig. 5. Element geometry around a vessel in the FDM. Cross-section perpendicular to the vessel axis. The *dotted lines* give the lines along which the heat flow is calculated

ed. Figure 5 shows a cross-section perpendicular to the vessel. The shape of the new vessel with four boundary elements and the surrounding elements is defined by the directives of the finite difference theory (Croft and Lilley 1977). The heat balances can now be made for the whole new geometry, thus calculating the temperatures at time $t+t$ from the known temperature distribution at time t. By repeating this step, the transient temperature distribution can be followed. A detailed description of the incorporation of discrete vessels in finite difference thermal models is given in Lagendijk et al. (1984).

Results

With the computational model described, we can calculate the thermal equilibrium length for every vessel type. To find this equilibrium length, we calculate the temperature rise in vessels entering a heated tissue volume. The introduction of the variable $u = x/<v>r^2$, with x being the coordinate along the vessel, makes possible a general plot of the temperature rise for every laminar flow vessel as a function of u. This general description of the temperature rise of laminar flow vessels has been confirmed by our thermal model by various simulations of different vessel types. In Figure 6, the general plot is given both for a laminar flow vessel entering a "muscle" tissue and for a laminar flow vessel entering a "fat" tissue volume. From this plot we find that the thermal equilibrium length for vessels in "muscle" tissue is given by: $X_{eq} = 9 \times 10^6 <v> r^2$ and in fatty tissues by $X_{eq} = 25 \times 10^6 <v> r^2$. In Table 1, the thermal equilibrium lengths for some specific vessel diameters and velocities are given.

Of the three vessel-type phases, Phase I represents the large vessels with equilibrium length that are much longer than the actual physiological length of these vessels (Table 1). This implies that no thermal equilibrium exists between the blood in these vessels and the surrounding tissue. These vessels must be considered individually in thermal models and they are the main cause for the inhomogeneous temperature distributions measured in

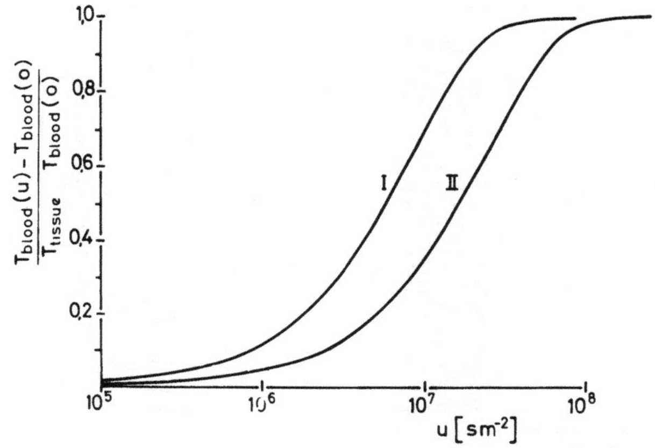

Fig. 6. General plot of the relative heating of laminar flow vessels entering a "muscle" tissue volume *(I)* and a "fat" volume *(II)* with temperature T_{tissue}. $u = x/<v>/r^2$; x is the coordinate along the vessel, and $x = 0$ at the location where the vessel enters the heated area

Table 1. Data of the vascular system of 13-kg dog (Mall 1888; Green 1950). Thermal equilibrium length for muscle tissues

Name	Diameter (mm)	Number	Length (cm)	Velocity (cm/s)	Xeq (cm)
Aorta	10	1	40	50	11250
Large arteries	3	40	20	13.4	270
Main branches	1	600	10	8	18
Secondary branches	0.6	1800	4	8	6.5
Tertiary branches	0.14	76000	1.4	3.4	0.15
Terminal arteries	0.05	1000000	0.1	2	1.1 10^{-2}
Terminal branches	0.03	13000000	0.15	0.44	8.9 10^{-4}
Arterioles	0.02	40000000	0.2	0.32	2.89 10^{-4}
Capillaries	0.008	1200000000	0.1	0.07	1.0 10^{-5}
Venules	0.03	80000000	0.2	0.07	1.4 10^{-4}
Terminal branches	0.075	13000000	0.15	0.07	8.9 10^{-4}
Terminal veins	0.13	1000000	0.1	0.3	1.14 10^{-2}
Tertiary veins	0.28	76000	1.4	0.8	0.14
Secondary veins	1.5	1800	4	1.32	6.7
Main veins	2.4	600	10	1.48	1.92
Large veins	6.0	40	20	3.6	2.92
Vena cava	12.5	1	40	33.4	11740

clinical practise. Figure 7 gives a calculation example of the inhomogeneous temperature distribution in tissue caused by the cooling influence of one large artery and one large vein running through an area heated with a uniform absorbed power distribution.

If these large vessels run through an area that is relatively small in comparison with their thermal equilibrium length, they can be replaced by heat sink lines of the actual body core temperature in the model. This simplifies the computer calculations.

Phase III describes the very small vessels with thermal equilibrium length that are much smaller than their actual physiological lengths (Table 1). No temperature difference exists

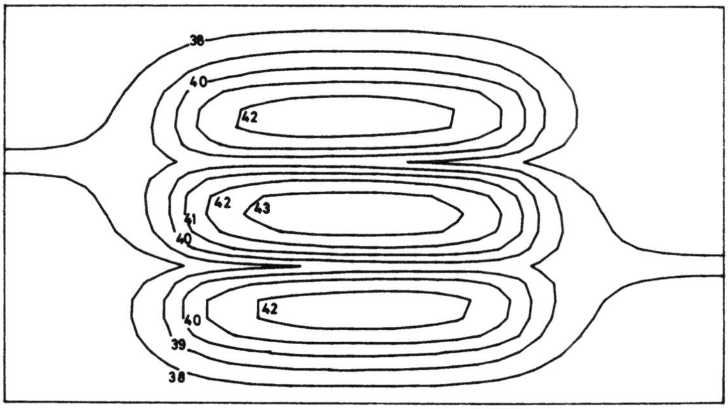

Fig. 7. Isotherm plot of the temperature distribution in a tissue block (18 × 12 × 6 cm) with an area (8.5 × 7.5 × 4 cm) heated with a uniform absorbed power distribution (P= 14.5 W/cm^3). The area is crossed by one large artery and one large vein (both: $<v>$ = 2.0 cm/s, r= 0.14 mm). Distance between the vessels is 3.0 cm

between these vessels and the surrounding tissue temperature. The relatively little influence of these thermally insignificant vessels on tissue heat transport can be taken into account by introducing an effective thermal conductivity K_{eff3} (Chen and Holmes 1980). As it is spatially variable and mostly temperature dependent, K_{eff3}can easily be taken into account in finite difference thermal models.

The intermediate Phase II is of extreme importance. Most heat transport in tissue is related to the blood flow in these Phase II type vessels. If the venous vessels are ignored, this phase causes the introduction of the "bioheat transfer" heat sink term B. In local hyperthermia, Phase II arteries, along with the large Phase I arteries and veins, cool down the local tissue volume. However, if the venous Phase II vessels are considered, these vessels now act as a source of heat for the local tissue volume. The venous vessels cool down and thus deposit heat in the local tissue volume. This venous heat source term can compensate for the arterial heat sink term.

The heat transfer process in Phase II falls between the collective description of Phase III and the individual description of Phase I. However, the Phase II vessels are too small to be taken into account individually in thermal models. These models will become too complex, for the anatomical blood vessel network data is not available. To solve the Phase II problem, we have to make the following realistic assumptions: (1) veins follow the same pathway as arteries, for they have a reverse flow direction, and (2) arteries and veins are of the same size at the same location.

According to these assumptions it follows that the arterial heat sink and venous source terms would cancel each other out (counterflow heat exchange), provided the vessels are small enough and are located close enough to each other. The remaining influence on heat transport of these Phase II vessel pairs can then be described by a greatly increased effective thermal conductivity K_{eff2}. At present, calculations are being carried out using our numerical model to find the relations among vessel diameter, mean blood flow velocity, distance between the vein and artery of the vessel pair and the vessel packing density, and the effective conductivity describing the vessel pairs.

Figures 8-10 give an example of these calculations. Figure 8 shows the model geometry, Fig. 9a gives the stationary temperature distribution in the tissue block without vessels,

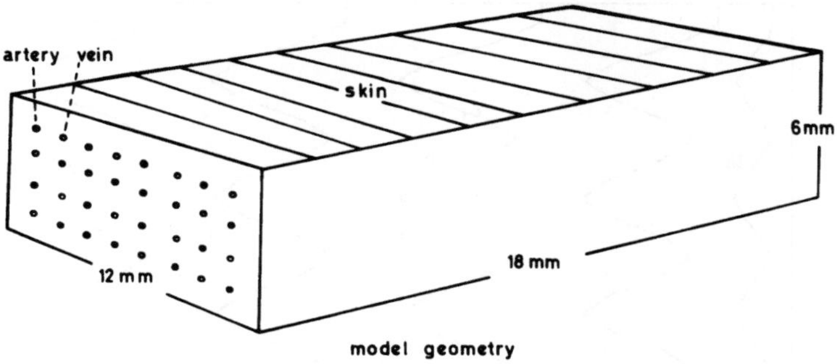

Fig. 8. Model geometry. The "muscle" phantom block 36 × 18 × 12 mm, with a thermal conductivity of 0.6 W m^{-1} K^{-1} and a specific heat of 4.2 J 9^{-1} K^{-1}. The block contains 32 vessels each with a diameter of 0.48 mm and a flow velocity of 1.5 cm/s. The initial block temperature is 37 °C. From time $t=0$ the left side of the phantom is kept at 44 °C, the right side at 37 °C. The other sides are thermally isolated

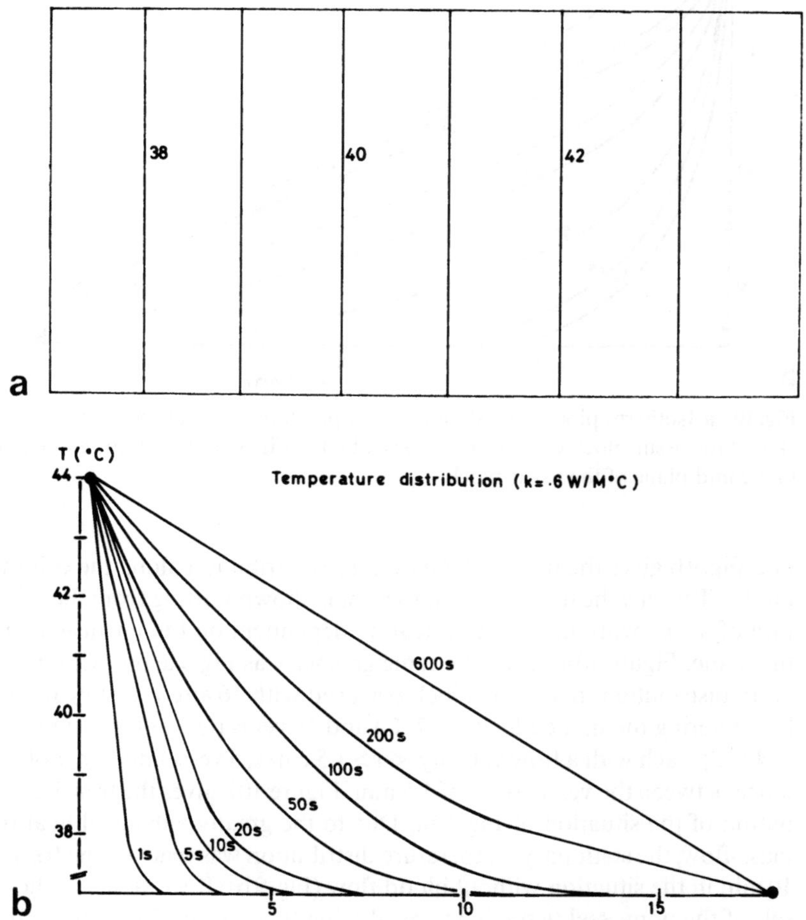

Fig. 9. **a** Isotherm plot of the stationary temperature distribution in the mid-plane parallel to the skin of the tissue block without vessels. **b** Transient temperature distribution along the central axis through the mid-plane for the situation without vessels

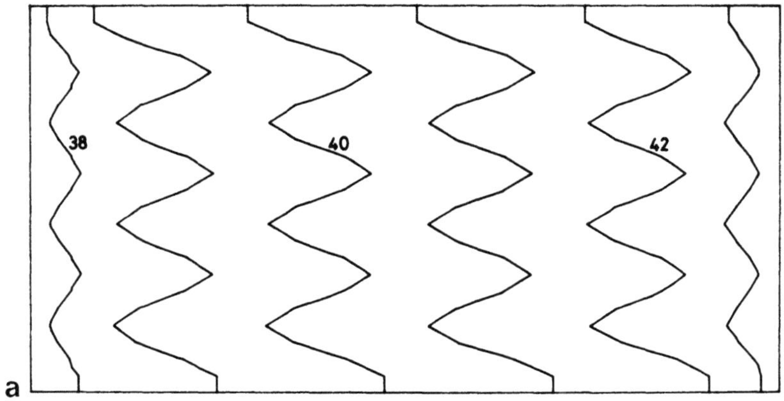

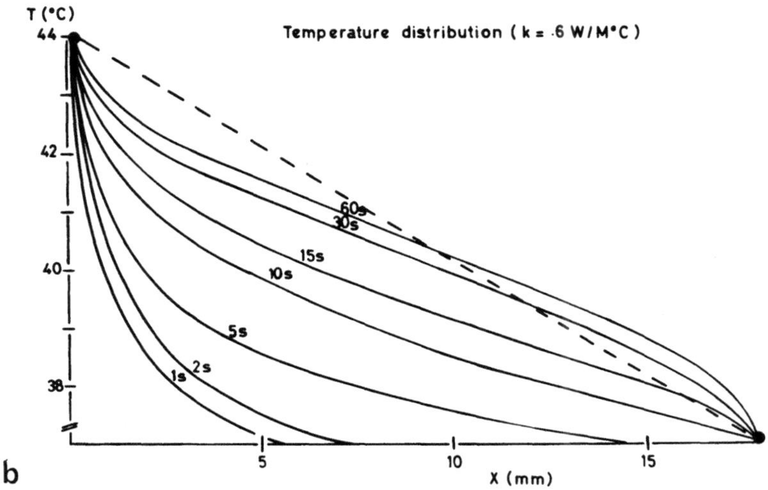

Fig. 10. a Isotherm plot of the stationary temperature distribution in the mid-plane parallel to the skin of the tissue block with vessels as described in Fig. 8. **b** Mean transient temperature distribution in the mid-plane of the tissue block

and Fig. 9 b gives the transient temperature distribution along the central axis through the model. The slow heating from left to right is shown starting from the initial tissue temperature of 37 °C, with the speed of heating dependent on the intrinsic thermal diffusivity of the tissue. Figure 10 a shows the same geometry as Fig. 9 a, but with the stationary temperature distribution in a tissue block perfused with 16 arteries (flow direction from right to left, entering the tissue block at 37 °C) and 16 veins (left to right, entering the tissue block at 44 °C), each with a flow velocity $<v>$ 1.5 cm/s, a vessel diameter of 0.48 mm, and a distance between the vessel pairs of 1.5 mm. Figure 10 b gives the transient temperature distribution of the situation of Fig. 10 a. Due to the greatly enhanced heat transport by blood mass-flow, the stationary temperature distribution was reached in 60 s, in comparison with 10 min in the situation without blood flow (Fig. 9 b). If we simulate the situation with vessels of the nonvessel tissue block by altering thermal conductivity of the tissue (K_{eff2}), we find that this vessel group can be described by a K_{eff2} of 7.2 W m^{-1} K^{-1} (Fig. 11). The temperature distribution shown in Fig. 10 is slightly disturbed by the limited size of the model and the boundary conditions selected. By describing the discrete vessels by an effective

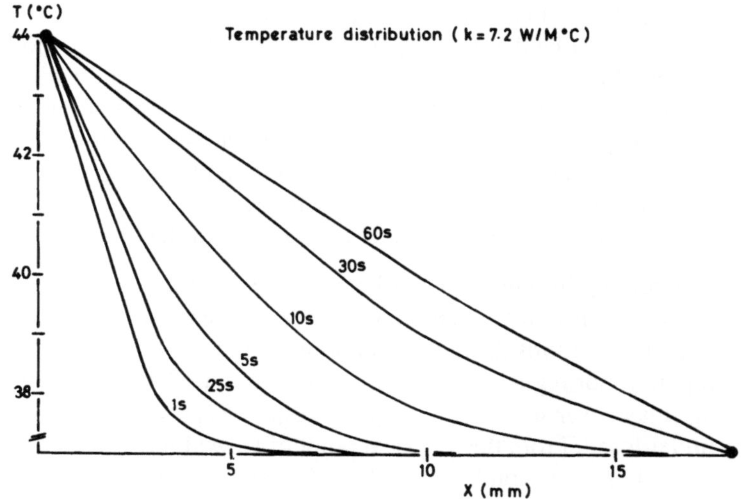

Fig. 11. Transient temperature distribution along the central axis through the mid-plane now without vessels but with the vessel influence simulated with an effective thermal conductivity of 7.2 W m^{-1} K^{-1}

thermal conductivity the temperature distribution is smoothed. This implies that, depending on vessel type, details of temperature distribution are lost.

Extensive simulations have to be done to find the effective thermal conductivity for all Phase II vessel pairs. The fine structure in the temperature distribution is directly related to the borderline drawn between Phase I and Phase II vessel types. Increasing the fine structure of the model makes the model much more complex and requires a larger amount of physiological blood flow data. Shifting the borderline toward the larger Phase I vessels simplifies the model and decreases the amount of anatomical data necessary, but leads to a loss of information on the actual small-scale temperature distribution in tissue.

Conclusions

Heat transport in tissues is dominated by its relation to blood flow. The influence of blood flow is characterized by the cooling effect of large vessels and the enormous heat transport, described by an effective thermal conductivity, of the Phase II and Phase III vessels. The heat transport due to this effective thermal conductivity is much higher than the heat transport due to the intrinsic thermal conductivity of the tissue (Figs. 10, 11).

Influence of the large vessel and the Phase II and III effective thermal conductivity rules out the conventional "bioheat transfer" theory, which entirely neglects the significant influence of blood flow on heat conduction in tissues and the (cooling) influence of the large vessels.

The finite difference model allows a detailed investigation of the different heat transport phenomena in tissue. Extensive calculations have to be made to determine:

1. The borderline between Phase I and Phase II vessels, which is of extreme importance for the final complexity of the model
2. The K_{eff2} describing the heat transport due to the different vessel pairs

There is a danger in the sole use of the enhanced effective thermal conductivity in thermal models to describe the influence of blood flow. If the thermal model used does not incorporate the Phase I large vessels, the temperature distribution will be smoothed out by the high thermal conductivity. The actual temperature distributions measured in clinical hyperthermia practise are found to be nonuniform due to the influence of the large vessels. Thus it is essential to incorporate also the Phase I large vessels in thermal models when using the enhanced effective thermal conductivity.

We now notice two important clinical results of the thermal modeling described:

1. The cooling influence of the Phase I large vessels, which have a thermal equilibrium length that is much longer than the heated area, causes thermally underdosed areas. If such a vessel runs through a tumor area, underdosed tumor cells are inevitable, resulting in tumor regrowth if the tumor is treated with hyperthermia alone. This underdosage may cover such a volume (Lagendijk 1982) that even hypoxic tumor parts might be underdosed. From this physical point of view alone, we must argue that in cases where hyperthermia is combined with radiotherapy and a uniform temperature distribution cannot be guaranteed, the radiation dose must be as high as possible to kill hyperthermically underdosed tumor cells. This implies that in treatments with a curative intention hyperthermia must be provisionally considered as an addition to the standard radiation treatment, with the main goal of killing as many radioresistant parts of the tumor as possible and of reducing the amount of cells to be killed by radiotherapy, thus increasing the chance of tumor cure.
2. Because of the heating of the arterial vessels by the venous vessels leaving the heated area (counterflow heat exchange) temperature uniformity greatly increases if we increase the heated tissue volume.

In the case of inoperable breast tumors, for example (Hofman et al. 1984), temperature uniformity increases if all venous blood leaving the breast is heated. The arterial blood entering the tumor region is thus preheated. By heating the entire breast and not only the tumor region, a better temperature uniformity might be obtained. Damage to normal tissue by overheating must, of course, be avoided.

References

Bakker CJG, Vriend J (1984) Multi-exponential water proton spin-lattice relaxation in biological tissues and its implications for quantitative NMR imaging. Phys Med Biol 29 (5): 509-518

Bowman HF (1981) Heat transfer and thermal dosimetry. J Microwave Power 16: 121-133

Chen MM, Holmes KR (1980) Micro-vascular contributions in tissue heat-transfer. Ann NY Acad Sci 335: 137-151

Croft DR, Lilley DG (1977) Heat transfer calculations using finite difference equations. London Applied Science, London

Drew TB, Hottel HC, McAdams WH (1936a) Trans Am Inst Chem Eng 32: 271-305

Drew TB, Hottel HC, McAdams WH (1936b) Proc Chem Eng Congr World Power Congr. London, vol 3, pp 713-745

Green HD (1950) Circulatory system. In: Glasser O (ed) Medical physics, vol II. Year Book Medical Publishers, Chicago

Hand JW, Ledda JL, Evans NTS (1982) Considerations of radiofrequency induction heating for localised hyperthermia. Phys Med Biol 27: 1-16

Hofman P, Lagendijk JJW, Schipper J (1984) The combination of radiotherapy and hyperthermia in protocolized clinical studies. In: Overgaard J (ed) Hyperthermic oncology, vol 1. Taylor and Francis, London, pp 379-382 (Summary papers)

Hynynen K, Watmough DJ, Mallard JR (1981) The effect of some physical factors on the production of hyperthermia by ultrasound in neoplastic tissues. Radiat Environ Biophys 18: 215-226
Iskander MF, Turner PF, DuBow JB, Kao J (1982) Two-dimensional technique to calculate the EM power deposition patterns in the human body. J Microwave Power 17: 175-185
Jain RK, Grantham FH, Gullino PM (1979) Blood flow and heat transfer in Walker 256 mammary carcinoma. J Natl Cancer Inst 62 (4): 927-933
Lagendijk JJW (1982) The influence of bloodflow in large vessels on the temperature distribution in hyperthermia. Phys Med Biol 27: 17-23
Lagendijk JJW (1984) A new theory to calculate temperature distributions in tissues, or why the "bio-heat transfer" equation does not work. In: Overgaard J (ed) Hyperthermic oncology, vol 1. Taylor and Francis, London, pp 507-510 (Summary papers)
Lagendijk JJW, Schellekens M, Schipper J, van der Linden PM (1984) A three-dimensional description of heating patterns in vascularised tissues during hyperthermic treatment. Phys Med Biol 29: 495-507
Mall F (1888) Die Blut- und Lymphwege im Dünndarm des Hundes. Königlich Sächsische Gesellschaft der Wissenschaft. Abhandlungen der Mathematisch-Physischen Classe 14
Ozimek EJ, Cetas TC (1982) Thermal dosimetry during hyperthermia. Natl Cancer Inst Monogr 61: 509-512
Pennes HH (1948) Analysis of tissue and arterial temperature in the resting human forearm. J Appl Physiol 1 (2): 93-122
Strang R, Patterson J (1980) The role of thermal conductivity in hyperthermia. Int J Radiat Oncol Biol Phys 6: 729-735
Strohbehn JW (1982) Theoretical temperature distributions for solenoidal-type hyperthermia systems. Med Phys 9: 673-682
Van den Berg PM, de Hoop AT, Segal A, Praagman N (1983) A computational model of the electromagnetic heating of biological tissues with application to hyperthermic cancer therapy. IEEE Trans Biomed Eng 30 (2): 797-805

Temperature Field Computation for Radiofrequency Heating of Deep-Seated Tumors

R. Sonnenschein and J. Groß

Firma Dornier System GmbH, An der Bundesstrasse 31, 7759 Immenstaad/Bodensee, FRG

In autumn 1984, a publicly funded, long-term clinical research study will be started on the efficacy of hyperthermic treatment of the collum and bronchus carcinoma, the applicator being a capacitive heating device at the fixed radiofrequency of 13.56 MHz. As part of this project, the authors will be working on computational methods to determine locally the temperature distribution within the patient's organs, which, as is well known with deep heating, represents a difficult calculational challenge. Even though it is too early at present to give any quantitative details, a number of theoretical aspects have already been considered and will now be briefly discussed.

With deep tumor sites, temperature field calculations are viewed as a valuable, indeed indispensable, aid in hyperthermic therapy. During treatment preparation (therapy planning), they assist in selecting or even developing the proper treatment procedure. During hyperthermia application, moreover, a detailed and precise knowledge of the tissue temperatures is needed to adjust the irradiation device parameters dynamically to deliver an optimal heating pattern within the tumor region (temperatures within the therapeutic range, no cold spots left), while at the same time eliminating the risk of necrosis in the healthy regions (no hot spots allowed). As actual temperature measurements can usually only be made at a few isolated locations, numerical calculations are strongly desirable for overall coverage of the temperature distribution.

In view of the high precision required, crude modeling of the complex tissue structure, e.g., in two-dimensional geometry with simplifying assumptions, appears to be inadequate. It is therefore intended to describe the truly three-dimensional architecture of the patient's body as realistically as is computationally possible, even though this may place a heavy burden on the numerical side.

The given calculational problem naturally divides into two parts:

1. Determination of the heat release in a lossy dielectric from capacitive irradiation with monochromatic electromagnetic waves of 13.56 MHz
2. Computation of the temperature distribution within the irradiated tissues, once the heat production is known

Both subproblems are weakly interconnected through the slight temperature dependence of the heating rate; this nonlinearity can be easily handled by an iterative procedure (a few iterations will suffice).

Capacitive Heat Input. With a capacitive heating device, the patient is situated in the high-frequency electromagnetic field between paired metallic plate electrodes (applicators),

Recent Results in Cancer Research. Vol 101

each of which is usually not larger than a stretched hand. Since in this arrangement the lossy dielectric medium is in the near field of a transmitter/receiver, the behavior of the electromagnetic field near the electrode surfaces must be taken into account. The problem will not be solved by idealizing assumptions like scattering of an incoming plane wave, with the reflected wave portion satisfying a radiation condition.

Instead, the spatial distribution of the electric field vector on the electrodes will, as a first step, be given as a boundary condition. This open boundary problem may be closed by the following procedure: around the relevant part of the patient's body and also enclosing the applicators, the "problem space" with volume V and closed surface S is defined. On S the electric field formally satisfies a boundary integral equation, whose unknown kernal function (Green's function) reflects the field behavior outside V. In principle, the problem space may be chosen at will. Practically, however, it is given as a compromise; for numerical reasons, V should be taken as small as possible, whereas only with a large V may the desired level of accuracy be attained (an error in Green's function will then be of negligible consequence to the field solution inside the dielectric).

Since the patient is so close to the radiating electrodes, the electric field vector $\mathbf{E}_0$ on the applicator is itself influenced by the field distribution as a whole and, therefore, can be estimated only approximately. So the boundary condition $\mathbf{E}_0$ should be improved by iteration.

As may be easily seen, the calculational procedure just described requires enormous numerical capabilities (machine capacity and number of operations) so that realistic field evaluations could be prohibitively expensive. Clearly, approximations of some sort will be needed. Within the lower frequency range of up to 20 MHz, the quasistatic approximation allows a much simpler field representation, which will be described in more detail.

In the quasistatic approximation (also: approximately of long wavelength), which is exact for frequencies $F \to 0$, the rotational part of the electric field vector $\mathbf{E}$ is totally neglected, the electric and magnetic field components now decouple, and $\mathbf{E}$ is given as the gradient of a real scalar potential. The absorbed power density is written as:

$$P = \sigma (\text{grad } \Phi)^2 \tag{1}$$

Conforming with this model picture, the radiating electrodes are represented as equipotential surfaces, i.e., Φ is given there as a boundary condition $\Phi = \Phi_0$; the value Φ_0 is determined from the radiation power output of the applicators. Again, introducing a problem volume V with closed surface S (cf. Fig. 1), the potential Φ satisfies on S the boundary integral equation:

$$\Phi(\mathbf{x}) = 2 \int_S \{ g_0(\mathbf{x},\mathbf{x}') \frac{\delta \Phi(\mathbf{x}')}{\delta n'} - \Phi(\mathbf{x}') \frac{\delta g_0(\mathbf{x},\mathbf{x}')}{\delta n'} \} \, d^2x', \# \in S \tag{2}$$

The scalar Green's function $g_0\,(\mathbf{x},\mathbf{x}')$ in quasistatic approximation (suffix o) mirrors the field behavior in the outer region, comprising every object in the treatment room that might influence the electric field distribution, as well as the screening effect of the Faraday cage. A rather simple estimate, valid in vacuum surroundings, is:

$$g_0(\mathbf{x},\mathbf{x}') = \frac{1}{4\pi} \cdot \frac{1}{|\mathbf{x} - \mathbf{x}'|} \tag{3}$$

At points in V the potential satisfies

$$\Phi(\mathbf{x}) = \pm \Phi_0, \mathbf{x} \text{ on the electrodes} \tag{4}$$

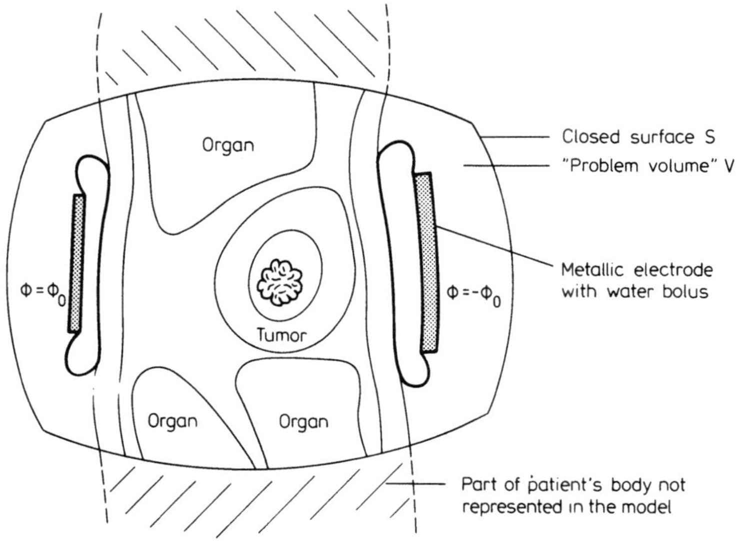

Fig. 1. Model configuration of radiofrequency heating applicators around patient's body with central tumor. In the electric field problem solution only the relevant part of the body, enclosed by surface *S*, is finely resolved

and otherwise the Laplace equation

$$\operatorname{div}(\varepsilon \cdot \operatorname{grad} \Phi) = 0 \tag{5}$$

Since the problem space is thought to contain regions with complicated geometrical structures, the finite element method is viewed as the most suitable numerical solution procedure. To this end, the differential equation formulation is transformed into an equivalent variational principle with the functional:

$$W|\psi| = \int_V \{\varepsilon(\operatorname{grad} \psi)^2\} d^3x - 2 \int_S \frac{\delta\psi}{\delta n} \psi d^2x \tag{6}$$

Making this functional stationary (in fact minimal) under the boundary conditions (2) and (4), the uniquely defined solution function Φ will be determined. This is approximately accomplished by the *Ansatz:*

$$\Phi(\mathbf{x}) = \sum_k \Phi_k f_k(\mathbf{x}), \# \in V$$

$$\varepsilon(\mathbf{x}) \frac{\delta\Phi(\mathbf{x})}{\delta n} = \sum_k \mathrm{h}_k f_k(x), \# \in S \tag{7}$$

The $f_k(x)$s are a class of preselected basis functions. The common choice is polynomials with only local support (= subvolume or finite element V_k) to which singular functions may be added to represent special features of the potential distribution in the vicinity of a metal edge.

From the stationarity postulate $\delta W|\Phi| = 0$ and the boundary conditions (2) and (4), the following system of linear equations for the unknown coefficients $\Phi = \{\Phi_i\}$, $h = \{h_r\}$ is derived (McDonald and Wexler 1980)

$$\begin{pmatrix} S & G \\ C & Z \end{pmatrix} \begin{pmatrix} \Phi \\ h \end{pmatrix} = \begin{pmatrix} B \\ 0 \end{pmatrix} \tag{8}$$

with elements of system matrices and right-hand side given by

$$\begin{aligned}
S_{i,j} &= \int_V \varepsilon(\operatorname{grad} f_i) \cdot \operatorname{grad} f_j \, d^3x \\
G_{i,r} &= \int_S f_i f_r \, d^2x \\
C_{i,r} &= \frac{1}{2} G_{i,r} + \int_S f_i(\mathbf{x}) \int_S \frac{\delta g_0(\mathbf{x},\mathbf{x}')}{\delta n'} f_r(\mathbf{x}') d^2x' \, d^2x \\
Z_{r,s} &= - \int_S f_r(\mathbf{x}) \int_S g_0(\mathbf{x},\mathbf{x}') f_s(\mathbf{x}') d^2x' \, d^2x \\
B_i &= - \sum_{\mathbf{d}} S_{i,d} \Phi_d
\end{aligned} \tag{9}$$

The suffixes i, j refer to internal free element nodes (within V), r and s refer to surface nodes (on S), while d means a Dirichlet node on the applicator for which the value Φ_d is given ($\Phi_d = \pm 1$ say).

Special care is exercised when evaluating the surface integrals C and Z as they contain the singular function g_0.

Subdividing the problem volume into a large number of finite elements (fine triangulation) results in large but sparsely populated matrices. For such systems of equations, special computing algorithms are known (Wexler 1979).

The overall procedure has already been successfully applied (in a rather crude version) to a problem with axial symmetry, simplifying it to two-dimensional geometry (Hermeking 1983). With three-dimensional problems and particularly in cases of high-precision requirements, a substantially larger number of degrees of freedom (10^4–10^5) has to be dealt with. Therefore the most efficient computing techniques available must be put to use.

Heat Transport in Tissue. The adequate description of heat transport in living, blood-perfused tissue has been attemated in a number of publications over the past years. A fully satisfactory (both from the theoretical and practical points of view) method, however, has not been found.

The problem essentially consists of the correct representation of blood perfusion, which has been proved to be quite significant for tissue temperatures. To be specific, a complex architecture of vasculature (Fig. 2), on the periphery of a rapidly growing tumor, say, may be envisioned.

Two classes of blood vessels can be distinguished:

1. Through big arteries, fresh blood, of basal temperature T_A, is transported into the tumor region at a high rate. Owing to their large heat capacity, these vessels may absorb a large portion of the heat input from the surrounding tissue, resulting in a local temperature dip there that could be therapeutically unacceptable. Clearly this effect is less important the smaller the vessels are.

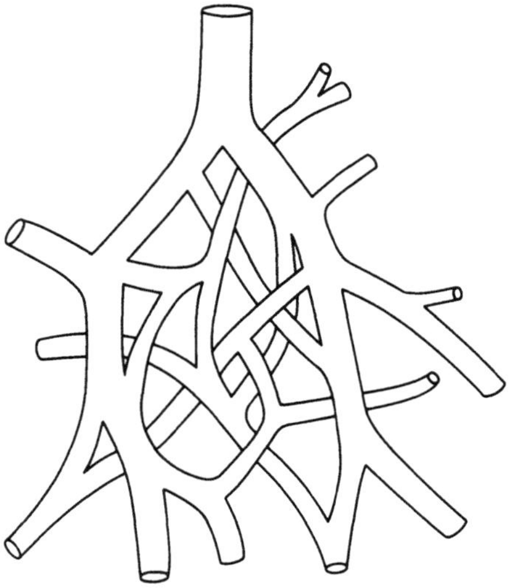

Fig. 2. Sketch of three-dimensional complex architecture of local macrovascular network

2. Blood vessels of medium and small size are so numerous and are interconnected in such a complicated network that there is practically no way of detecting them individually or representing them all in a numerical model. For temperature determination, moreover, their exact representation appears to be quite unnecessary, as they rather quickly equilibrate with the tissue. Thus this microvasculature is best dealt with in a continuum picture.

Depending on the degree of complexity in modeling the perfusion, different forms of heat transport equations are arrived at. The simplest formulation, the bio-heat equation, is:

$$\rho c \frac{\delta T}{\delta t} = \mathrm{div}\,(\lambda\,\mathrm{grad}\;T) + \rho \cdot \rho_{\mathrm{B}} C_{\mathrm{B}} W_{\mathrm{B}} \cdot (T_{\mathrm{B}} - T) + Q \qquad (10)$$

A suffix B refers to blood; the other variables are for tissue containing blood where some volume-averaging has to be understood. λ is the true conductivity (without convection), T_{B} the global arterial base temperature, and Q the heat production density from metabolism and electromagnetic irradiation. All quantities, with the exception of T_{A}, may be position and temperature dependent. Of particular variability with temperature is the specific perfusion rate W_{B} (measured, e.g., in ml/min 100 g), since it reflects the ability of the organism to react upon an environmental heat input.

The bio-heat equation is relatively easy to tackle by numerical computation. Its solution, however, only halfway solves the problem of determining the local tissue temperature, because as a volume-averaged quantity (the averaging procedure is not clearly defined) T does not necessarily show local extrema (cold and hot spots).

The bio-heat equation will therefore be sensibly employed for a rough first estimate of the tissue temperature distribution on the whole. While in special cases it may provide rather exact temperature results, in general the quality of the computed temperature field is not expected to be sufficient.

Taking the heat exchange processes with large vessels into account individually could mean a considerable improvement over the bio-heat equation. A systematic analysis leads to the following heat transport equation for tissue (Chen 1982):

$$c\rho \frac{\delta T}{\delta t} = \operatorname{div}(\vartheta + \vartheta_B) \operatorname{grad} T + \rho_B c_B \cdot \{\rho W_B (T_B - T) - \mathbf{U}_B \cdot \nabla T\} + Q \tag{11}$$

Heat transfer by microcirculation is approximated by an increase in the heat conduction current (div ϑ_B grad T), an additional convection current ($-\rho_B C_b \mathbf{U}_B \cdot \nabla T$) as well as a perfusion term [$\rho \cdot \rho_B C_B W_B (T_B - T)$] with changed parameters W_B, T_B, which are now position dependent. W_B stands for the specific local perfusion rate of the medium-sized and small vessels which should be determined experimentally; T_B is their local arterial entrance temperature and is to be computed simultaneously with the microvolume-averaged tissue temperature T. This quantity agrees more closely with the true local tissue temperature, first, with increasing blood vessels are represented individually and, secondly, with better knowledge of local heat exchange processes with large vessels.

Exactly where the borderline (limit resolution) between large and small blood vessels should be drawn for a particular organ under study cannot now be answered generally. At any rate the structure of the vasculature of the tumor and its surroundings should be closely inspected and carefully modeled in each individual case (it is supposed that measurement of the macrocirculation is possible and therapeutically justifiable).

Of course, modeling the vascular network with increasing complexity and detail very soon leads to a computational limit beyond which a solution is no more feasible. An analysis by Lagendijk et al. (1983) shows that even for comparatively simple systems (which are still not representative of deep-seated tumors), the numerical effort will be enormous. It is expected though that, taking advantage of every special computational trick, it should be possible to refine further the theoretical description of blood perfusion to a sufficiently high degree that systems of much more complicated architecture (e.g., like the one in Fig. 2) may be realistically evaluated. Because of its truly three-dimensional geometry, finite elements appear to be best suited. The relatively large regions of the body that will be heated (tumor together with subcutaneous fat and bones) with deep heating devices result in a high number of nodes, as is the case with the electric field subproblem.

References

Chen MM (1982) Mathematical modelling of heat transfer in living tissues - the formulation. In: Nussbaun GH (ed) Physical aspects of hyperthermia. AAPM Monogr 8: 549-564

Hermeking H (1983) Temperaturfeldberechnung zur Hyperthermiebehandlung. BMFT-Forschungsbericht T 83-268

Lagendijk JJW (1984) A three-dimensional description of heating patterns in vascularised tissues during hyperthermic treatment. Phys Med Biol 29 (5): 495-507

McDonald BH, Wexler A (1980) Mutually constrained partial differential and integral equation field formulation. In: Chari MVK, Silvester PP (eds) Finite elements in electrical and magnetic field problems. Wiley & Sons, New York

Wexler A (1979) Perspectives on the solution of simultaneous equations. Dept of Electrical Engineering, University of Manitoba, Canada

Summary and Conclusion

Physical Point of View

J. W. Hand

Medical Research Council, Cyclotron Unit Hammersmith Hospital, Ducane Road,
London, W12 OHS, United Kingdom

The question as to which regions of the human body may be heated adequately using currently available techniques can be answered as follows. Superficial tumours at depths of 3-4 cm can be heated and their temperatures controlled reasonably well using microwave methods or low-radiofrequency methods. Ultrasound methods may produce heating at slightly greater depths. Our ability to heat deep-seated tumours, however, must be looked at more pessimistically. Several groups are investigating this very difficult problem. There are many physical and physiological problems, which must be carefully studied if we are to progress with electromagnetically induced regional heating. If deep localized heating can be induced by ultrasound, concurrent improvements in thermometric techniques will be required. However, interstitial methods are capable of heating rather large volumes relatively uniformly and are applicable to both superficial sites and those deep in the body. A further advantage is that many of these methods can be combined with interstitial brachytherapy.

In the fields of thermometry and thermal modeling there have been several interesting proposals as to how the considerable problems which exist might be solved. Ideally, we need a noninvasive thermometry system which is adaptable to all regions of the body. All the methods currently being investigated (using velocity of ultrasound, T_1 relaxation in NMR, CT numbers) are in their initial stages. Microwave thermography is applicable in superficial sites of depths of 2 or 3 cm. There is no system available that makes it possible to use this method for deep regions.

Invasive thermometry will remain the basis of thermometry for some time. Progress has been made in the area of nonperturbing probes using optical fiber technology, and the availability of multisensor probes is increasing. The single-sensor thermometer reported at this workshop, based on the Fabry-Perot principle and a temperature-dependent frequency shift, appears to be better in accuracy and stability than those thermometers currently available measure intensity.

Theoretical aspects of thermal modeling are progressing well. The fundamental problems involved are recognised and detailed two-dimensional models of regional hyperthermia are being set up. However, these are in the early stages of development and, whilst useful for comparing techniques, do not yet allow real treatment planning. Similarly, at present there is no way of accurately predicting temperature distributions in patients.

Recent Results in Cancer Research. Vol 101

Clinical Point of View

H. D. Kogelnik

Institut für Radiotherapie, Landeskrankenanstalten Salzburg, Müllner Hauptstrasse 48,
5020 Salzburg, Austria

In the search for improvement in local tumor control, several biological experiments and early clinical results have established a definite advantage for hyperthermia therapy.

The need for an additional measure is demonstrated by some figures: at present 35%–40% of patients can be cured, using all treatment modalities: surgery, radiation therapy, and chemotherapy. The remaining 60%–65% of patients can be divided into two groups: about two-thirds die as a result of distant metastases and one-third die of the primary tumor, i.e., the local or the locoregional disease cannot be treated adequately.

In order to improve local control rates and to prevent metastases, hyperthermia is beginning to be introduced into the therapy schedule. Of the new programs that have been started in this field, hyperthermia seems to be one of the most promising.

Recent Results in Cancer Research. Vol 101

Subject Index

MIX
Papier aus verantwortungsvollen Quellen
Paper from responsible sources
FSC® C105338

If you have any concerns about our products,
you can contact us on
ProductSafety@springernature.com

In case Publisher is established outside the EU,
the EU authorized representative is:
Springer Nature Customer Service Center GmbH
Europaplatz 3, 69115 Heidelberg, Germany

Printed by Libri Plureos GmbH
in Hamburg, Germany